Arthritis Diet & Plant Based Nutrition

universal. As befitting its nature, it is presented without assurance regarding its prolonged validity or interim quality. Trademarks that are mentioned are done without written consent and can in no way be considered an endorsement from the trademark holder.

BONUS:

As promised, please use your link below to claim your 3 FREE Cookbooks on Health, Fitness & Dieting Instantly

tiny.cc/o2u27y

You can also share your link with your friends and families whom you think that can benefit from the cookbooks or you can forward them the link as a gift!

Table of Contents

Arthritis Diet:

Anti-inflammatory Diet for Arthritis Pain Relief

Chapter 1: Introduction

Congratulations on purchasing the *Arthritis Diet* and thank you for doing so.

If you have purchased this book, it's possible you or a loved one have symptoms of arthritis and joint pain. Maybe you even have inflammation and been diagnosed with an inflammatory disease. If that's the case, we can understand how hard that is for you, and we sympathize with you. This book is a great introductory read to learn about the symptoms of joint pain and arthritis, as well as how inflammation affects the body. It explains these conditions so you can become familiar with them and can easily recognize symptoms that might be plaguing you. Whether you are experiencing pain, stiffness of the joints, or having limited motor function, arthritis can affect every individual differently. It can be a struggle trying to figure out how to work around the pain as your normal daily routine is interrupted. Whether you are elderly or not, arthritis can require a change in lifestyle, maybe limiting the activities you once did regularly and getting in the way of an active lifestyle.

This book will also touch on the possible causes of arthritis. Though there is some research to prove that rheumatoid arthritis can be genetic and linked to certain genes, not all arthritis types occur this way. If someone in your family like your parents or siblings have arthritis, you are more likely to have the disease too. But arthritis itself can manifest in many ways depending on the lifestyle you are living. People who have extremely physical jobs such as professional athletes or stunt performers may develop arthritis at a younger age due to the impacts on their body. Even people who perform manual labor jobs and are constantly repeating the same gestures or movements throughout their workday can have arthritis occur at those joints. Along with lifestyle, your medical history also plays a role. If you have had previous bone injuries, even with the proper treatment and healing time, it's possible that the bone and cartilage did not repair itself well. In fact, it's impossible for the repair to ever be like it was before, and any fracturing or tiny indentations can make the bone vulnerable to future breaks. People who have also battled with viral or bacterial infections, such as meningitis or staph infections, also are vulnerable due to their weakened and more fragile bones. Due to this, they may find themselves plagued with joint pain and arthritis earlier in their life.

When it comes to arthritis and inflammation, you're probably wondering what you can do to heal these aches and pains. Part of it is a natural degradation of the body, but there are many treatment options that can work to ease discomfort. Medication has advanced by leaps and bounds. Whether you're simply taking over the counter medication or stronger narcotics, it's important you first have a medical exam conducted and speak to your primary care physician about your individual care of pain. There are also individualized therapies that you can regularly attend. Whether you participate in traditional therapy, water therapy, or an exercise class, it's important that exercise and an active lifestyle becomes a part of your life, so your joints do not become even more brittle from lack of use.

This book touches on changes you can make to your diet to hopefully reduce your arthritis pain and or inflammation flare-ups. The research strongly indicates that having a balanced diet full of a variety of foods is most healthy for people battling arthritis. The more variety you consume, the more you are naturally ingesting different vitamins and minerals that your body may be lacking. Most of the time, the body processes these nutrients much better as a food item instead of over the counter vitamin supplements! Taking a pill might sound easier, but adding a vitamin or nutrient to your meals could provide you with the better benefits.

It's important to have fruits, vegetables, dairy, and grains in your diet. Each group of food provides a variety of vitamins and fiber to make your bones strong. When it comes to adjusting your diet, it's also necessary to cut out the sugary and salty processed snacks. Instead, try adding healthy snacks into your diet like beans, nuts, or yogurt. These are all proven to be very filling and may even help if you are trying to lose weight. Yogurt is even considered a superfood because it contains so many probiotics that can help your digestion! We also provide more than a dozen delicious smoothie recipes that consist of only healthy ingredients that fight against inflammation. These treats are so delicious, that you won't even remember all the health benefits associated with them! It's as simple as gathering your ingredients and pulsing your blender for a few minutes!

We hope this book is helpful to you and answers your questions on a healthy diet to reduce symptoms of arthritis and inflammation. Thank you for reading!

Chapter 2: What are Arthritis and Inflammation?

If you suffer from arthritis and joint inflammation, you most likely are already familiar with the terms and key concepts behind them. For other readers, this chapter will provide an introduction into what exactly these conditions are.

Inflammation is a necessary part of the body's healing process. You may remember from high school biology that the body's white blood cells and immune system cells work in the immune system to fight off bacteria and infection for us. Inflammation occurs naturally when the body is fighting off infection. But with some diseases, the body's immune system triggers an inflammatory response even when there is no infection to fight against. These diseases are collectively called autoimmune diseases and can be very detrimental. Because the body mistakenly turns on itself and fights against normal, healthy tissue, it can greatly damage a person's system if not properly diagnosed and treated.

Arthritis is a term commonly referring to inflammation of the joints or the tissues that sound the body's joints. Arthritis itself refers to almost 200 conditions in the medical spectrum. Types of arthritis that are more commonly known are rheumatoid arthritis (RA), osteoarthritis, fibromyalgia, or lupus. Common symptoms of arthritis can involve stiffness, swelling, or pain in the joints or around the joints, but certain forms of arthritis, like lupus, can affect the body's organs and wreak havoc on the body as a whole. According to the Centers for Disease Control and Prevention (CDC), more than 50 million Americans have some form of arthritis. Although this condition is commonly associated with the elderly, it can affect people of all ages, even young children depending on what ailment they may have been diagnosed with.

Arthritis can be a range of symptoms, and it differs on how it affects an individual person in their day to day activities. Some people can experience severe pain in their joints and feel their routine is severely affected, limiting their movements and activities. Severe arthritis can make it even hard for you to lift your arms and legs. Those who have limited symptoms may be able to fight past the twinging of their knuckles or swelling they feel. There can be a decreased range of motion the more arthritis develops, along with symptoms of pain, swelling, and redness at the joints.

Rheumatoid arthritis is classified as an autoimmune disorder, or a disorder where the body turns on itself and attacks its own tissues. The body's immune system attacks the joint capsule, which is a hard membrane that covers and protects all the joints in our body. The lining becomes inflamed at the attack and a person will experience the common symptoms of swelling and pain at the joints. This disease is a complex one to diagnose because it can start so innocently with just some slight pain or swelling in the hands or wrists. We might pass it off as the usual type of aches and pains. But rheumatoid arthritis is a progressive disease. If the disease progresses without treatment, the body can even destroy the cartilage and bone within the joint. The inflammation can spread to other parts of the body and cause a severe disability. If early symptoms are noticed and seem to be getting progressively worse, a doctor will perform the necessary exams and tests to determine if and how badly the joints have been eroded. This type of arthritis seems to run in families and research has found it tied to two genetic markers. Smoking also seems to exacerbate this arthritis. Environmental factors like obesity, stressful events, and exposure to viruses or bacteria can also cause an individual to develop rheumatoid arthritis.

Juvenile idiopathic arthritis is a type of rheumatoid arthritis that affects children. According to 2015 Census data, nearly 1 in 2,000 children have this disease. If a patient has been diagnosed before the age of 16, it's counted as juvenile arthritis. Due to the young age, this disease can be even harder to identify in young adults so doctors may look at their medical history to see if they have battled any other diseases or infections. Juvenile cancer patients will tend to have this arthritis due to the weakness of their bones. Nearly 10% of juvenile arthritis patients are systemic that affect the entire body with symptoms like fever, limping, and swelling, and stiffness of the joints.

Osteoarthritis is the most common degenerative form of arthritis especially in the elderly. According to the Centers for Disease Control and Prevention, more than 30 million Americans are affected by this disease. This type of arthritis does not have inflammation as a major role in it. Neither do arthritis types such as fibromyalgia or common muscular back or neck pain. But rheumatoid arthritis, gout, and lupus are all arthritis diseases associated with inflammation in the joints. This means the inflammation of the joints does not stay localized and instead can damage other joints or the underlying bone, even turning on the body's muscles and other organs.

Although childhood arthritis is not as common, juvenile arthritis can still occur especially in children who have been exposed to bacterial or viral infections. They tend to show symptoms a lot earlier due to these infections and may have had lasting permanent damage to their joints. Sadly, there is no cure, but if caught and treated early, symptoms can be managed and contained through medication and therapy. If symptoms are noticed and do not get better, it's important a doctor do a complete medical exam to assess any damage and degradation to the joints.

Inflammation is a natural process of the body that occurs to fight diseases, infections or pathogens that are trying to attack the body. The immune system gears up for an attack on any invading cells and the body uses inflammation to fight any chemicals or irritants. Acute inflammation, or inflammation that is only temporary, is normal and a sign of a healthy body fighting back. For example, if you've cut your finger, you might feel a swelling sensation there, and the area looks red and puffy. That's a sign your body is sending cells into overdrive to heal the wound. But when the inflammation begins to occur without any infection or wound, that's a sign the body is getting mixed signals. Chronic inflammation that occurs for a long period of time can even damage internal organs if not treated. There are different inflammatory diseases that can affect the heart (myocarditis), kidneys (nephritis), eyes (iritis), and even the muscles and blood vessels (vasculitis). It can occur at multiple sites and can be tragic if caught too late. Inflammation in the lungs is very serious too and can lead to conditions like asthma and bronchitis. When the lungs become inflamed, the airways become constricted and breathing becomes more difficult. Imagine if you had just finished running a race or working out, and how you are panting for breath. With inflammation of the lungs, patients' breathing can become agitated like that without even working out or exerting themselves.

Symptoms of inflammatory arthritis do not only occur at the joints. Patients can experience other major symptoms and it's important that they are diagnosed as soon as possible. Along with pain in the joints, there could be other body pain and constant fatigue as the body tries to fight back against the inflammation. The treatments involve a combination of exercise and medication to help patients reduce the pain that is affecting their lives. Gout and lupus are two common forms of inflammatory disease. Lupus can affect so many parts of the body like the wrists, knees, and hands.

Inflammatory arthritis can be especially debilitating because it affects so many parts of the body. Along with the physical pain, a person can experience psychological stress as they cope with their symptoms and lack of body control. People in the workforce may have to leave their job due to the pain and go on disability. It's important that along with medicine and physical therapy, patients also have access to mental health resources as they adjust to the changes in their life. Often serious diseases linked to inflammation and arthritis can cause depression, mood disorders, or insomnia. A 2015 study published in JAMA Psychiatry found that patient with depression had more than 30% brain inflammation. Education on the disease and counseling from a licensed therapist are resources your doctor's office can often prescribe you. It is also beneficial to have a good support system to help with making lifestyle adjustments and keeping patients upbeat and feeling positive.

The important thing to realize about having and living with arthritis is that your entire lifestyle needs to adapt to the disease. As you are adjusting your lifestyle to cope with the pain and stiffness of your joints, you should take positive steps to maintain your activity and healthy eating habits to combat your symptoms.

Moderate exercise has been shown to be helpful in managing the pain. Losing weight might also be something your doctor recommends if you are carrying extra pounds that are putting stress on your joints. Eating a healthy diet consisting of lots of fresh fruits and vegetables is also important. This book will provide information about which foods can help combat symptoms of arthritis and inflammation. If you've successfully cut out salty or sugary snacks from your diet, we can provide you with some great ideas of what to start eating instead, like nuts and granola. Even adding some simple ingredients to your food preparation steps like ginger, garlic, turmeric powder, and using extra virgin olive oil can help you gain the beneficial properties these foods offer.

Chapter 3: The Causes of Arthritis

There are many risk factors associated with arthritis. Some types of arthritis do run in families, and you can be more likely to develop arthritis if your parents or siblings also have it. Research on rheumatoid arthritis has found it linked to genetic markers called HLA-B27 and HLA-DR4. A study of the HLA antigens in 105 unrelated American Caucasian patients with rheumatoid arthritis found that HLA-DR4 was observed in 71% cases that showed a familial trend of rheumatoid arthritis. It was also found in 63% of the non-familial cases. This correlated with another similar experiment conducted on Scandinavian patients in Finland that also found high frequencies of DR2, DR3, and DR4 in arthritis patients. These studies have allowed the scientific community to state that familial occurrence of rheumatoid arthritis could lie in these genes. If a relative has presented with the condition, then it is much more likely to show up again in the family tree.

Other types of arthritis seem to be less influenced by genetics and can be a result of other factors. Older age is the most common mark for arthritis patients because the human body's cartilage naturally becomes more brittle as we age. The older we get, the harder it is for our body to repair itself. Osteoarthritis is known as the common "wear and tear" on the body's joints and mostly occurs in individuals between 40-60 years old. Depending on other risk factors and lifestyle choices, it can even manifest itself earlier. Women are more likely than men to develop osteoarthritis though the research is not clear why that is the case. Other autoimmune diseases, like gout, tend to run higher in males.

Obesity is also a high-risk factor when it comes to developing arthritis. Those who suffer from obesity are carrying excess weight for their joints to manage, and that adds stress to the weight-bearing joints, such as the knees, spine, and hips. The extra weight greatly impacts the joints in those areas and the inflammation that occurs can gradually wear away the joint tissues. Research states that for every extra pound of weight gained, your knees gain three pounds of stress! When it comes to hips, the ratio becomes one pound of weight to six times the pressure on the hip joints! Fat tissues also can produce proteins that cause inflammation around the joints. People who have excess body fat can find themselves struggling with pain and tenderness in their joints much earlier than someone who is not obese. The cartilage at the junction of the joints begins to break down a lot earlier due to the excess weight that has become a burden to your body. That is why one of the first things a doctor will prescribe to an overweight patient exhibiting signs of arthritis is weight loss. Implementing a healthy lifestyle that promotes weight loss can sometimes help people reduce their symptoms of arthritis. They may notice a difference in their symptoms and more relief than before they had the extra pounds.

Additional risk factors to getting arthritis include previous injuries or having had infections during some point in your life. When a joint is previously broken, it can repair itself unevenly despite the injury seeming to be healed. This is especially true for sensitive areas like the wrist and the knee joint. Previous bone injuries can impact the complex structure of the bone and cartilage, so it does not react the same when faced with compression or impact. You may have heard stories of someone breaking their wrist and then many years later due to a fall or car accident, breaking it again in the same spot. This is due to the injury spot becoming more vulnerable after it was healed. It cannot hold up to a second point of impact or compression. The same is true for certain bacterial or viral infections that can affect the joint and cartilage regions. People who experience a joint infection or a staph infection have those areas of the joints deteriorated and run a higher risk for developing arthritis even after the infection has been treated. Even after the injury has healed, the cartilage repair is never the same as it once was before the injury. There could be flaws in the healing process. The damage to the joints stays and symptoms of arthritis can begin to show earlier in these patients' lives.

It's also important to understand how certain lifestyle choices can bring a higher risk of arthritis. People who tend to live a lifestyle of high sports activity or extreme physical activity can experience symptoms of arthritis earlier, such as professional athletes, stuntmen, etc. It's not only people who play contact sports, such as football or wrestling, but also sports that place repeated stress on the joints such as cycling or long distance running. The repeated activity over a period of time can break down the joints and the cartilage slowly and cause an athlete to develop arthritis even if they are not yet close to the age when arthritis usually occurs. On the reverse side, moderate exercise tends to minimize the symptoms and can actually give a muscle more strength and buoyancy. Doctors will encourage patients to implement a short exercise routine into their day to alleviate the pain and swelling in their joints. It's the repeated, long-term activity that people may be taking part in during an eight-hour a day shift at work that can cause damage. This includes even minor movements like pushing a cart or typing at a keyboard. That's often why jobs that involve manual labor or repetitive movement urge employees to stop often for breaks as a preventative measure to try and minimize damage. These employees are urged to walk around or stop their repetitive movement for at least 15 to 30 minutes every few hours to give the body a break and give those joints some relief from the repeated stress.

Despite these risk factors and environmental conditions, it's important to realize that arthritis itself is a common condition and one that scientists believe that all humans will one day afflicted with. It's only natural given the wear on our bodies and how fragile we become as we age. Whether there is a family history or not, arthritis may be a condition we all battle with in our future and one we see our elderly loved ones living with now. The next step is to educate ourselves about this disorder so we may recognize the signs and get help as needed. Whether it's medication, physical therapy, or additional supplements, your body will need help to fight this disease. Incorporating healthy eating habits into your life may be able to provide some pain relief, or at least slow the degradation of your bones as you accumulate more vitamins and minerals.

Chapter 4: Understanding Inflammation and Arthritis

In order to properly understand inflammation and the resulting joint pain, it's important to understand how the body's immune system uses inflammation in a normal way. As we discussed briefly in Chapter 1, the body's immune system composed mostly of white blood cells works to fight off infection and bacteria. It is a part of the body's healing process as cells work in overtime to fight against an infection. It's a defense system set up by our body to protect itself and white blood cells are the first line of attack. When attacked, either by an infection or an open wound of some kind, the white blood cells quickly receive growth factor hormones and send nutrients to the affected area. They swoop in and fight the infection and ingest other foreign radicals in the area. Swelling happens naturally because the movement of the blood cells and hormones to the area brings with it fluid as well. That's why the nerves at the area become so sensitive to touch.

When inflammation occurs naturally due to fighting off an infection, it's because the body releases chemicals into the bloodstream or at the affected tissues. These chemicals increase blood flow to the area and the area can turn red or warm. Sometimes the chemicals can leak fluid around the tissues and that's when swelling occurs. The nerves at the area become overstimulated and the area becomes very sensitive to touch. Have you ever noticed this when you've had an injury? The area can feel like it's burning or itching, and you can't help but feel a tingling sensation as if you want to scratch. That's because, at the localized area of the injury, cells are working together in overtime to heal you. It's the same function that occurs when you have a sore throat. The inflammation in the area is due to the body fighting against an infection. This is called acute inflammation which is simply the body reacting to a foreign agent or wound. Usually, once the infection has passed, the swelling will go away and the area will become normal again.

With inflammatory arthritis, the inflammation occurs for no reason. There is no infection or injury present that needs healing - it's simply the body turning on itself and causing the symptoms of inflammation to occur. Those symptoms such as pain, stiffness, and swelling, start affecting an individual in their daily activities and use of the joints. Eventually, the increased activity at the joints can wear down the cartilage at the bones and even cause the lining of the joints to swell. The inflammation can even begin to occur at the site of major organs, such as the eye, kidneys, lungs, or heart. Symptoms of inflammation need to be assessed immediately with a complete medical history and physical exam conducted. Other tests like X-rays and blood tests should also be studied to assess how far the damage has progressed, and if there is any way to reverse it. This type of persistent long-term inflammation is called chronic inflammation and many autoimmune disorders fall into this category. Asthma, allergies, inflammatory bowel disease, lupus, Crohn's disease... all these fall in the category of diseases with chronic inflammation. The body mistakenly sends signals to the organs to become inflamed even though there is no threat. The white blood cells arrive at the area and find no threat, so they begin attacking the body's own cells and tissues.

It's hard to imagine the scientific phenomenon of pain, but the sensation of pain is the body's response to warn us regarding an injury. In the case of arthritis, there is an injury to your joints which the body is becoming aware of and is sending out alert signals about. The damaged tissue around the joints releases neurotransmitter chemicals that carry the message up your spinal cord and to your brain. The brain processes the signal it received and sends a signal back to your motor nerves to respond. For example, when you cut yourself, the message is instantly sent to your brain and you move your hand away.

It's important to note that the commonly known ailments of muscle pain and back pain are not necessarily tied to arthritis and joint pain. Soft tissue pain is felt in the tissues rather than the joints. It tends to occur when parts of the body are overused repeatedly, or due to an injury. Back pain can be due to many factors, such as damage to the nerves, bones, joints, muscles, or ligaments. If these symptoms are temporary and can be relived easily enough with medication or a massage, they would not fall under the category of chronic inflammation which continues to occur for a longer period of time.

Chapter 5: How to Manage Arthritis Pain

The good news is that science has progressed rapidly to battle the types of arthritis discovered. These diseases are often diagnosed correctly now instead of simply passed off as "creaky old bones", especially in elderly patients. Non-inflammatory types of arthritis can often be treated with over the counter pain medications. Often a lifestyle change, such as weight loss, and a routine of physical activity can help to relieve symptoms.

In fact, doctors will often prescribe physical therapy to help elderly or sedentary arthritis patients become gradually more familiar with physical activity. This is especially true for elderly patients who are finding it hard to be mobile and need a push to incorporate an exercise regime into their lifestyle. Individual physical therapy is geared specifically for what the patient needs and what is the best remedy for their condition. Whether it's arm joint pain or knee pain, your therapist would work with you to create a routine to exercise the affected joint area. Sometimes a therapist may also use massage techniques, or use ice or heat packs to relieve pain.

Water therapy is also a great form of specialized therapy that can provide ease for patients. Water supports an individual's weight and puts less pressure on the muscles and joints. It provides resistance to your muscles which in turn exercises them and makes them stronger. This is very helpful for patients who might be overweight and just beginning to exercise. It gives a person, especially an older person, a buoyancy and lightness to help them feel more agile than they may have in years! Many people mistakenly think of aquatic exercises as swimming or diving, but that's not the case. Instead, these are simply exercises that are performed while the person is standing in water that is about waist or shoulder level. Regularly performing aquatic exercises can help relieve pain in patients and improve the movement in their hip or knee joints.

Therapy can be something you pay for or is prescribed by your doctor if you need more specialized care, but regular old fashioned exercise is something any doctor will recommend. (Keep in mind, this varies case to case because someone's arthritis may be more severe or coupled with other illnesses.) Exercise is considered one of the best ways to manage pain in osteoarthritis patients. Their pain can even be reduced if they regularly exercise. Walking is one of the best ways to exercise without adding too much stress on the joints. As an aerobic exercise, it also strengthens the heart and lowers blood pressure. In arthritis patients specifically, it tones the muscles that support joints in the body, and as you age, it can slow the loss of bone mass. Studies have found that people who have arthritis but who participated faithfully in an exercise routine were less likely to need hip replacement surgery compared to arthritis patients who did not exercise. The patients who exercised even reported having overall better physical health and more flexibility and range of motion.

There are a few types of exercises that are recommended for arthritis patients to help ease their pain and the stiffness in their motions.

- Flexibility exercises: These exercises refer to the range of motion a patient may be having difficulty with. For example, the joint is not moving to the full motion that it used to before. Maybe someone is having knee pain where they cannot stretch their leg as they used to before. Flexibility exercises focus on gently stretching and expanding the range of movement at that joint. A therapist may first show you what type of exercises to perform and how to stretch the joint and the surrounding muscles, but these exercises can easily be performed in the comfort of your home without help. Performing them regularly can help flexibility return in those joints. It's like the old saying goes - practice makes perfect! You may not get back complete range of motion, but it may certainly be better than before.

-

- Strengthening exercises: These exercises work to strengthen the muscles. Strong muscles work to protect the joints in the body. The stronger your muscles are, the more cushion they can provide joints that are affected by arthritis. Strengthening exercises can be done with a medium to light range of weights, and ones that can be attached to your feet to strengthen leg muscles. These exercises should also be done many times a week to continue to exercise the muscles and build endurance.

-

- Endurance exercises: These are also called aerobic exercises because they strengthen the heart muscle. These exercises include things like walking, bicycling, swimming, or using the elliptical or treadmill machine. Activities like this build up a person's stamina and make their lungs more efficient. Not only that, but it also provides physical exercise for the whole body, allowing you to stretch and exercise many joints, muscles, and ligaments.

When it comes to deciding how often you should exercise, it's important that each patient follow their physical therapist or doctor's advice. Generally, flexibility or range-of-motion exercises should be done every day to help the joint become familiar with the new stretches. Other exercises should be done for a minimum of 20 minutes a few times a week, but it all depends on how vigorous the exercise is performed. It's also important that patients be aware of their own arthritis and the fragility of their condition. Depending on age, the severity of the disease, and range of motion, your activities should fit your abilities and your lifestyle. For example, someone elderly with severe arthritis should be playing a high impact sport, but stay limited to their flexibility exercises. Someone younger may still be able to jog or swim a few times a week to keep their joints and muscles strong and their heart healthy. Arthritis patients will want to be move slowly and carefully in their routine as to avoid any fractures or injuries. Always be sure to warm up and cool down with enough stretching time before and after working out to properly relax your muscles!

There are many categories of medication that also assist with joint pain and inflammation. There are non-steroidal anti-inflammatory drugs that reduce pain and inflammation. These tend to be available over the counter, such as Advil, Motrin, and Aleve. They are even available as creams or patches to be applied to the problem area for ease. This is great for traveling, or to have applied if you will be sitting for a long period of time. Analgesics is a category or medication that can reduce the pain of arthritis but will not affect inflammation. Tylenol, or acetaminophen, is available over the counter, but narcotics like Percocet, Oxycontin, or Vicodin can only be prescribed by a doctor. Before a patient progresses to stronger drugs that contain oxycodone or hydrocodone, he or she would need to have battled arthritis for a longer period of time and not found relief with alternative methods. Because these drugs have addictive properties, their use would need to be carefully monitored by a doctor.

For arthritis associated with inflammation, disease-modifying antirheumatic drugs work to stop the immune system from attacking itself and the joints, or at least slow down the attack. These medications are prescribed to rheumatoid arthritis patients. Corticosteroids suppress the immune system and work to reduce inflammation at the sight of the pain. Patients with more serious inflammation disorders that are classified as autoimmune disorders would need to be monitored carefully with regular testing and doctor's visits.

As we mentioned in the previous chapter, obesity is also a risk factor for arthritis. Because of this, it makes sense that one of the first things that a doctor would prescribe to an obese patient is weight loss. The more excess body weight you are carrying, the faster the progression of arthritis can occur as well. The cartilage at the joints begins to wear down faster as a result of the excess weight it has been carrying. Losing weight can reduce the stress on the joints. People will often notice an ease in their arthritis symptoms when they lose a significant amount of weight and maintain a lifestyle that keeps the pounds off. They begin to feel better physically and experience a wider range of motion than they did before. This is simply to state that a patient should not be offended if they are recommended to lose weight by a doctor. The research shows that it will be beneficial in the long run.

Chapter 6: Healthy Eating Habits

To follow a routine of eating healthy to combat your arthritis, it's important to be aware of what kind of diet you need to set. You should be sure to eat nutrient-rich foods and avoid sugary or fatty snacks that can cause inflammation or trigger weight gain that would further exacerbate your arthritis. Research suggests that the type of diet you are eating, coupled with whether you are exercising, can play a major factor in the progression of your disease and the symptoms you exhibit. There is no magic cure for these diseases, but a variety of foods and a balanced diet can benefit a person who has symptoms of arthritis.

Research regarding patients and dairy ingredients have come up inconclusive despite evidence showing both sides. A 2015 study in the Journal of Nutrition found that eating dairy foods increased inflammation in a group of adults selected for the sample. A similar study found that osteoarthritis patients who ate more dairy were more likely to need surgery for a hip replacement. On the other hand, numerous studies show that eating more yogurt and drinking more milk can lower the risk of gout, an autoimmune disease we mentioned earlier that also showcases arthritis. The conflicting evidence can leave patients torn about how to incorporate dairy into their daily diet.

Most research has painted dairy products in a positive picture. A recent 2017 study found that dairy does have beneficial anti-inflammatory effects except for in people who are allergic to cow's milk. Keep in mind that "dairy" does not just refer to milk, but also ice cream, cheese, and yogurt. There are many food items to consider in that category. The good news is that research on yogurt has come back consistently positive. The probiotics in it are associated with decreased insulin resistance and decreased inflammation in the body. Just like with any other diet, moderation is key. Overeating high-fat dairy products or sweetened products will not help in terms of weight loss which is also very important to minimize inflammation.

Some people find that avoiding certain foods can reduce their arthritic flare-ups. For example, if a certain type of milk is associated with negative symptoms, you can try an elimination diet and quit eating it for a while. This can show you how your body responds, and it's possible you feel better without cow's milk.

Another debate that has sprung up is the concept of organic foods. There is no strong evidence that supports eating organic food can minimize your chances of getting autoimmune diseases or arthritis. But it can make sense to minimize your exposure to unwanted chemicals by choosing an organic diet. When you eat foods that are from conventional farms that use hormones or chemicals, you're ingesting that as well every time you have eggs, meat, or cheese. But besides that, logical fallacy, there's no evidence that states conventional food is bad for people with arthritis. It's important that even if you are not buying organic produce, you still are consuming a diet full of a variety of fruits and vegetables. All fruits and vegetables should be washed thoroughly or in a water and vinegar rinse to remove any harmful pesticide residues. If you can afford it, try buying some organic produce, like the ones with soft exterior skins that you directly consume such as peaches, spinach, or bell peppers. The consensus by doctors has been that a serving of at least 5 fruits and vegetables a day is considered healthy for an arthritis patient. If you are concerned about possible pesticides or growth hormones, buying organic or non-GMO foods is a personal choice up to you.

Antioxidants in produce tend to fight inflammation and are also a major source of nutrients. Having a variety of fruits and vegetables gives you the ability to take in more vitamins and nutrients. Try to incorporate vegetables into your snacks more. For example, if you're having a sandwich, instead of just a slice of cheese or some low-sodium meat slices, add in some vegetables so you're getting a serving of produce as well. If you're planning on having a salad, try adding in some fruit or nuts to increase the proteins you're taking in, and surprise your taste buds!

When it comes to meat and seafood choices in your diet, fish is encouraged as it provides a great source of anti-inflammatory omega-3 fatty acids. It can be substituted easily for red meat in your diet, especially if you are at risk for high disease or have high cholesterol. If you are not familiar with where to start when it comes to choosing fish, there are dozens of varieties for you to choose from! If your local grocery store does not have many options, try finding a local fish market to find fresh options. Avoid processed meats that tend to contain preservatives and are high in sodium. Try to buy more lean cuts of meat with fat trimmed off. Turkey and chicken are also healthier substitutes to red meat.

Make room in your diet for whole grains like cereal and pasta. Instead of white rice that tends to be high in carbohydrates, try experimenting with alternatives like quinoa or wheat. You can even find pasta that are made of vegetables or chickpeas so that they are lower in starches and sugars. Be sure to read the ingredients when trying new items to be sure you are getting the protein you need, and that items are low in sugar and carbohydrates.

Try and cut out packaged and processed snacks from your diet. The sugar and salt content in these products cause health concerns and are not helpful to a weight loss lifestyle. There are healthier alternatives out there that have their snacks based on vegetable or legumes instead, like lentil chips or roasted garbanzo beans. Be sure to read the label carefully when finding a new snack to make sure it's as healthy as it could be addictive! If your local grocery store does not have many healthy options, you may have to find a local organic grocery store or browse online to see what options are available. This also includes being careful of what canned foods you buy. You want to be sure you always drain the liquid in the cans and rinse the beans, or fruit, or whatever you are going to be eating. You want to be sure the fruits have preserved in their own juice, not in a sugary syrup that packs on calories. There are tons of canned beans and lentils out there that are easy to store and make to whip up a quick vegetarian recipe. Be sure that the sodium level is 5% or less per serving.

It's important to note that there is no research that proves abiding by a vegan or vegetarian diet could be the cure to inflammation. In fact, studies on this have been mixed. Some studies found that people who were strictly on a vegetarian diet had no alleviation of pain or stiffness in their joints compared to the control group that followed a traditional diet with meat. Other studies have found that patients who followed a vegan diet for months at a time tended to have improvement in their swollen joints and less stiffness in the morning compared to the control group. With these mixed results, doctors will not urge you to follow a vegan or vegetarian lifestyle. It is important to note though that a meat-free lifestyle can lead to lower cholesterol and blood pressure levels and decrease your chances of becoming obese. But there are also downsides to these diet choices.

Vegetarians, and especially vegans, tend to have lower levels of vitamins in their blood, as well as low calcium and fatty acids. These substances are crucial to bone health. Vegetarians also tend to have lower levels of HDL which is the "good cholesterol".

If you are considering making a major change in your diet plan to help with your inflammation or arthritis, it's important you first speak to your doctor about the risks and reasons. There are other ways you can reduce your meat intake such as adding a "Meatless Monday" to your weekly schedule or incorporating a side of vegetables or a salad more often. If you do decide to cut meat entirely from your diet, then your doctor may need to run a blood test to see if there are any vitamin supplements you should be taking orally.

Foods That Fight Arthritis

Although there is no direct cure for arthritis and it is really a balanced lifestyle of exercise, diet, and medication, some foods are believed to fight arthritis. Adding these items to your regular diet could ease your symptoms of inflammation. Here is a beginners list to what you should try and incorporate into your meals!

- Fish: Fish is a source of high protein and packed with omega-3 fatty acids that fight inflammation. Doctors recommend at least 3 to 4 ounces of fish consumed twice a week. Tuna, mackerel, herring, salmon... whatever your favorite is, try having it for dinner once or twice a week to get the nutrients you need.

- Tofu: If you're a vegetarian and do not have fish or meat as a protein source, soybeans such as tofu and edamame are great alternatives that can also provide omega-3 fatty acids. These

34

substitutes are high in protein but low in fat which makes them a great substitute.

- Extra virgin olive oil: This oil was considered a luxury in the past because it has medicinal properties similar to anti-inflammatory drugs. When battling arthritis, it's important to even be aware of the type of cooking oil we are using. Including olive oil, walnut oil, safflower oil, and avocado oil also have properties that can lower cholesterol and a high content of omega-3 fatty acids.

- Berries: Anthocyanins have been researched and found to have an anti-inflammatory effect and can reduce the frequency of gout attacks in patients with that autoimmune disorder. Along with these health benefits, anthocyanins tend to give fruits their rich purple or red color, like in cherries, strawberries, blueberries, and blackberries. The whole berry family!

- Dairy: Despite what we mentioned earlier about the studies conducted on dairy and arthritis symptoms, milk, cheese, and yogurt are all packed with Vitamin D and calcium which are essential for the body. They are both necessary to increase bone strength, so it's important they be consumed on a moderate basis. If you are lactose intolerant or have a dairy sensitivity, then you will have to search for substitutes that work for you. Leafy vegetables and lentils are a great substitute for those who may be allergic to dairy.

- Garlic: Studies have found that people who ate more foods from the allium family, like onions, leeks, and garlic, showed fewer signs of osteoarthritis. Raw garlic itself is found to have many health benefits like lowering blood sugar levels and regulating blood pressure. You want to try and consume it in its raw or semi-cooked form as much as you can though because it loses many of those properties once cooked. Garlic has been found to even block the presence of enzymes that damage cartilage in the body - which is great news for arthritis patients. So, mince some raw garlic and add it as a garnish on your soup or salad to gain the benefits it can provide!

- Broccoli: Broccoli is rich in vitamins C and K, and contains a compound called sulforaphane which researchers believe can slow the progress of osteoarthritis. It is also rich in calcium which is beneficial for building strong bones.

- Green tea: We've been hearing for years about the benefits of this drink and the antioxidants it provides the body. Researchers have studied the antioxidant epigallocatechin-3-gallate (EGCG) that stops the production of molecules that causes joint damage in patients with rheumatoid arthritis. If you've been an avid coffee drinker, try a cup of green tea instead!

- Citrus: Grapefruits, oranges, clementines... you name it! The citrus family is rich in vitamins and that works to prevent arthritis and maintain healthy joints in the body. Another great tip is to use fresh lemon or lime juice in recipes instead of the concentrated kind.

- Nuts: Nuts are one of those rare treats that are high in good fats, so they are considered "heart healthy", in moderation, of course. They also contain many beneficial vitamins like calcium, zinc, vitamin E, protein, and fiber. They are helpful if you are trying to lose weight because a handful of them can be very filling and allow you to cut back on the portions you're consuming. There are tons of options out there for you to find exactly which is the perfect nut for you. Pistachios, almonds, walnuts, pine nuts, macadamia nuts... it's all out there! Be sure that you are consuming these nuts in their raw form though. If you are leaning more toward the chocolate covered or salted version then you are canceling out the health benefits.

- Whole Grains: While most diets would urge you to stay away from carbohydrates, whole grains are unique because they provide the beneficial effect of lowering the levels of C-reactive protein in the blood. C-reactive protein tends to be found with signs of inflammation in the body and is associated with an increased risk of diabetes, rheumatoid arthritis, and even heart disease. Including things like rice, whole-grain cereals, and low-fat oatmeal in your diet is a terrific way to maintain low levels of this protein in your bloodstream. Research has shown that people who had fewer servings of whole grains in their diet tended to have higher inflammation markers. The fiber found in whole grains also helps with weight loss.

- Beans: Beans a great and inexpensive source of healthy vitamins and minerals such as zinc, potassium, iron, and protein. Beans and legumes are well known for the benefits they provide to the immune system. You don't have to create a fancy recipe if you don't know how to incorporate them into a meal - just have canned beans handy and add a handful to your salad or rice bowl. Kidney beans, pinto beans, and red beans are especially great to keep the heart healthy.

Foods That Fight Inflammation

As stated above, there is no direct cure for arthritis and it is all about managing a healthy lifestyle that includes your diet, exercise, and medication if needed. Researchers have found that a diet resembling a Mediterranean diet is actually very helpful to fight inflammation. This diet is comprised of lots of vegetables, fish, and using olive oil instead of a different type of oil in cooking. There are some foods that have proven to be beneficial and can combat symptoms of arthritis. Adding these to your regular diet could ease your symptoms. Here is a beginners list to what you should try and shop for and incorporate into your meals!

- Fish: As stated above, fish is a great alternative to red meat, especially in patients who are also battling high cholesterol or at risk of heart disease. Fish contains high amounts of omega-3 fatty acids that work to reduce the amounts of interleukin-6 and C-reactive protein (CPR) in the body. These two proteins are involved in creating inflammation in the body. Research encourages inflammation patients to have at least 3 to 4 ounces of fish twice a week. Whether it's tuna, sardines, salmon, herring, or mackerel... pick a type of fish that you enjoy the most and give it a place in your weekly menu. Grilled, smoked, fried... the options are endless!

- Colorful Fruits: Anthocyanins are antioxidants found naturally in colorful fruit such as raspberries, blackberries, cherries, and strawberries. It's also found in high amounts in leafy vegetables like broccoli, kale, and spinach. These work to naturally fight inflammation in the body. Be sure to incorporate at least 2 to 3 servings of fruits and vegetables in your day. It's all about having a variety of those fruits so you can naturally take in as many antioxidants as you can. Watermelon is especially beneficial because it contains choline, an inhibitor that blocks signs of inflammation in the body's white blood cell network.

- Nuts or Seeds: Nuts are great snack items that are full of monosaturated fat, or the "good fat" that works to fight inflammation in the body. On top of that, they're full of fiber and very filling. They're a great addition to your diet, especially if you're trying to cut back on how much you are eating throughout the day. This can work to fill you up, fight inflammation, and may even help you lose a few pounds! There are tons of healthy options for nuts so browse the snack aisle and see which your favorites are. There's walnuts, pistachios, almonds, or a healthy trail mix combination of all the above! Be sure that you are picking natural nuts without any additives or sugar or salt which would defeat the purpose of such a healthy snack. Try and eat a handful of nuts a day to fight inflammation and increase your "good" cholesterol levels.

- Beans: Beans are another substance that naturally have anti-inflammation compounds and are packed with antioxidants. And they're very cost efficient too! You can buy them already prepared in cans or buy a big bag to keep in your pantry. They are packed with lots of nutrients like folic acid, protein, iron, potassium, and zinc too. There are also many varieties out there so you can pick and choose which you prefer. Black beans, pinto beans, garbanzo beans, red kidney beans... we hope you have a favorite that you can incorporate into your diet at least twice a week.

- Olive Oil: There's a reason olive oil is sometimes referred to as "nectar of the gods". It contains heart-healthy monosaturated fats and tons of natural antioxidants that work to lower inflammation in the body. Just a few teaspoons used in cooking can be enough for you to gain the benefits of this miraculous oil. Extra virgin olive oil is less processed and contains even more nutrients than standard olive oil. It can be on the pricey side though, so you can save it for use on salads as a dressing or in soups. You want to be sure that when ingesting olive oil you are keeping it at low or room temperature. High heat destroys the structure of the polyphenols in the oil or the natural compounds that elicit the health benefits we described. Avoid using it for frying or baking, but be sure to incorporate it into your salad dressings or adding a little to your pasta before a meal.

- Fiber: Fiber is another excellent source that works to reduce inflammation in the body. It lowers the amount of C-reactive proteins (CPR) in the bloodstream (these are one of many proteins that cause inflammation). Research has found that ingesting fiber through food works better to lower CPR levels than simply taking over the counter supplements. Because of this, it's important that patients have a fiber-rich diet. Whether it's coming from vegetables (like potatoes, celery, or carrots), fruits (bananas, apples, and oranges) or from whole grains (like oatmeal or fiber-rich cereal), be sure you have a fiber-rich diet. You can also ask your doctor about adding a fiber supplement to your diet if you feel you aren't eating enough.

- Onions: Leeks, onions, garlic, and green onions... all these members of the allium family are linked to lowering inflammation in the body. Onions contain quercetin, a compound that inhibits histamines that cause inflammation, like when you have an allergy attack and your lungs become inflamed. They are packed with beneficial antioxidants and have many health benefits. Not only do they reduce inflammation, but also reduce the risk of heart disease and lower levels of LDL which is the "bad" cholesterol in the body. Try and incorporate onions into your meals, whether it's dicing them and adding them into your vegetables, grilling them with your meat, or including them in your pasta or sandwiches. If you don't like raw onions, you can always sauté them with a little seasoning - but go light on the salt and oil!

- Drink Moderately: Resveratrol, a compound found in red wine, is believed to have anti-inflammatory effects. So, sure, maybe a glass of red wine every now and again can have medicinal effects. But it is important to remember that people with rheumatoid arthritis should limit their alcohol intake, especially with higher dose medications. If you are a drinker, be sure to have a talk with your doctor about how much you are drinking and if it's okay with the medication you are taking.

- Avoid Processed Foods: We all know potato chips and other snacks in the junk food aisle are delicious, but the truth is, these snacks are not helping you gain any relief from inflammation. In fact, the additional salt in chips and other snacks can cause inflammation in the bloodstream as your body struggles to process the increase in sodium. In fact, a study at Yale University in 2013 showed an increased risk of having rheumatoid arthritis if they were more prone to a salty diet. This study has yet to be confirmed with more research but any doctor can confirm that extra salt is not a good thing for the body. An increase in processed foods can lead to weight gain which can increase your symptoms as your body adjusts to the more pounds you're carrying. Gaining a few pounds might not sound drastic to you, but the body's joints have to overcompensate for the new weight. Avoid these processed foods and try and stick with healthy snacks like nuts and whole grain granola for snacking.

Foods that Boost the Immune System

If you're looking into items that work to boost your immune system, here are some foods that researchers have found to have healthy benefits! It always helps to bolster your immune system and give you a better chance of fighting off infections. Though there are plenty of over the counter supplements, here are some items you can add to your diet to give you the same benefits.

- Citrus Fruits: Extensive research has shown that this family of fruits is loaded with high amounts of Vitamin C. This is especially necessary for the immune system because Vitamin C is believed to increase white blood cell production. White blood cells? Well, those are the first "soldiers" in the line of defense of your immune system to protect you against infections. Popular citrus fruits include grapefruits, oranges, tangerines, and clementines. Also, don't forget to use natural and organic lime and lemon juice whenever you can and in your cooking, as opposed to the ones from concentrate.

- Bell Peppers: Here's a fun fact - one ounce of bell pepper contains two times as much vitamin C as an ounce of fruit from the citrus family! Something about the color that gives this pepper its red quality also provides it with a stunning amount of vitamin C. These peppers also are packed with beta-carotene which keeps your skin and eyes healthy. With a beautiful selection of colors available, these are great to add to your salad or slaws. They add some color to your food and give you great health benefits too!

- Yogurt: Yogurt is a natural source of probiotics or "good" bacteria that live in your gut and help to digest foods. Not only that, but it also works to boost immunity. You want to be sure that you are avoiding heavily sweetened yogurts though because those tend to cancel out the positive health benefits. Try to find yogurts with fewer additives and be wary of ones that come packed with fruit. You can always add in your own fruit or granola to be sure you are getting all the health benefits!

- Ginger: Ginger is found to reduce inflammation and is perfect to reduce a sore throat or swollen glands if you are fighting off a cold. Just imagine having a hot cup of ginger tea when you're home sick with a fever! It's also been found to reduce nausea and lower cholesterol. If you are not able to eat a piece of ginger raw, have a mincer or zester handy so you can at least sprinkle some over your pasta or salads. Researchers at the University of Wisconsin found a few other spices that also have anti-inflammatory properties – oregano, cloves, nutmeg, and rosemary. If you're already a big spice lover, try and incorporate more of these into your recipes. If you're a newbie simply trying to gain the health benefits, experiment with these new flavors in your meals. You may find something delicious and healthy too!

- Chicken or Turkey: Along with all the other health benefits of white meat over red meat, chicken and turkey also contain high amounts of B-6 vitamins. Just 3 ounces of white meat contains nearly half your daily recommended amount! This vitamin is a very important part of the chemical reactions that occur in the immune system to form new red blood cells and keep them healthy. Chicken stock or soup that's made from boiling chicken bones also contains nutrients that help with immunity. There's a reason why they say chicken soup is the best medicine!

- Shellfish: Zinc is an important mineral that our body needs to instruct our immune cells how to function and which infections to fight. It's also very important in healing open wounds! Shellfish is a category of seafood that includes lobster, clams, mussels, and crab. Keep in mind that you want to have shellfish in moderate doses. Too much zinc in the bloodstream can inhibit the function of the immune system. Men should have about 11 milligrams a day, and women should have 8 milligrams.

- Tea: A Harvard study found that participants who drank at least 5 cups of black tea a day had nearly 10 times more interferons (proteins that signal amongst each other to fight viruses) in their bloodstream than participants who drank a placebo drink. L-theanine is an amino acid that is present in black and green tea. If you're already an avid tea drinker, try and stick to these types of tea. Be sure to get out all the nutrients you can from the tea bag before tossing it out!

- Garlic: Garlic naturally contains the ingredient of allicin which works to fight infections and bacteria in the body's immune system. A study in Great Britain found that out of 146 people given either garlic or a placebo for a period of 12 weeks, the ones given garlic were two-thirds less likely to catch a cold. Try and incorporate a clove or two of garlic in your meals, even if you're mincing it and adding it on top as a garnish.

- Eggs: We already know that eggs are a major source of protein, but they also are necessary for a healthy immune system. Eggs are rich in Vitamin D that is important for your bones. A deficiency in Vitamin D can increase your chances of upper respiratory infections during the winter, and even immune disorders like diabetes. Immune cells even have cell receptors that are constantly searching for vitamin D in the bloodstream! While you can get vitamin D through sun exposure as well, it's important that you are eating plenty of foods high in Vitamin D such as fish, beef, and eggs so that you are including it in your diet even in the winter season. Try and switch to a Vitamin D fortified milk too!

- Fish: We've been saying it repeatedly, but it's the truth - fish is packed with tons of omega-3 fatty acids that work to strengthen the immune system and potentially ease symptoms of arthritis and inflammation. Research has found that these fatty acids can fortify the lungs from a cold, reduce inflammation, and even protect you from the flu. Whatever type of fish you prefer (and there are tons out there to choose from!), be sure to have fish as a meal at least twice a week. For high cholesterol and heart disease patients, it's also a great alternative to red meat.

Vegetables to Include in Your Diet

If you're focusing more on which vegetables to shop for, here are some great suggestions that are full of beneficial vitamins and minerals. They might even help you strengthen your immune system if you are already fighting an illness, or simply trying not to get a cold this winter!

- Broccoli: We've heard it from childhood and that's because it's the truth - broccoli is good for your immune system. It has vitamins A, E, C, fiber, and natural antioxidants that work to strengthen the immune system. It contains high amounts of sulforaphane, an antioxidant that fights to reduce levels of NF-kB in your bloodstream. NF-kB is responsible for inflammation flare-ups in the body. The key to getting the most health benefits from broccoli is to cook it as little as possible. If you can eat it raw - even better! If not, lightly sauté it with a minimum amount of oil and seasoning. Other cruciferous vegetables that are associated with anti-inflammatory benefits include Brussels sprouts, cabbage, and cauliflower.

- Sweet Potatoes: Instead of the regular brown skin potatoes, sweet potato actually contains more beta-carotene which your body metabolizes into vitamin A that helps the immune system. Beta-carotene rich foods are identified easily by their bright orange pigment - sweet potatoes, carrots, squash, and cantaloupe. All are great sources to help your body intake vitamin A to help your immune system. A great way to enjoy your sweet potato is to load them with other healthy foods like a dollop of sour cream, a sprinkle of turmeric spice, herbs, and lemon or lime juice.

- Spinach: Another vegetable that haunts some us from our childhood dinner table, spinach is packed with lots of Vitamin C, and other antioxidants that help the immune system fight off infections. Like broccoli, the more raw you can consume it, the more health benefits you will gain. If you can have it added raw in your salad, that's the best option. But you can also sauté it lightly and have as a vegetable side.

- Mushrooms: The benefits of mushrooms have become more well-known in the last few decades and it's a well-deserved honor they're getting at the salad bar. Numerous studies show that mushrooms increase the production of white blood cells which is very helpful if you are sick or fighting a disease or infection. Reishi, maitake, shiitake mushrooms, and Portobello mushrooms have been found to help bolster immunity the most. Mushrooms are low in calories but high in vitamins, lectins, and phenols - all of which work together to fight against inflammation in the body. Whether it's on your pizza, sautéed as a side, or added to your pasta, be sure to include mushrooms in your diet when you can to get the benefits they offer. The less cooked you can eat them, the better it is for you to gain their full anti-inflammatory effect.

- Kale: There's a reason this vegetable is everywhere these days! Kale is a great source of vitamin A which works to strengthen your immune system in fighting off infections. Whether it's in a salad or a smoothie, or just added on as an afterthought in your pasta, try and incorporate a few servings of this in your diet throughout the week to get your recommended vitamin A intake. Like spinach that we mentioned above, leafy green vegetables like kale are a great source of anti-inflammatory agents. So whether you prefer spinach, kale, Swiss chard, or arugula, be sure to incorporate some of these greens into your diet!

- Tomatoes: Tomatoes contain high amounts of lycopene. Lycopene has been found to reduce the amount of inflammatory proteins in the bloodstream. A 2014 study even found that women who drank tomato juice regularly decreased their inflammation flare-ups. More helpful than taking lycopene supplements, ingesting raw tomatoes and tomato products are more helpful to reduce inflammation. It's important to note that lycopene is a fat-soluble nutrient, which means it's absorbed better by the body when it's paired with some fat at the same time. So, tomatoes are great to pair with some cheesy pasta, or added as a topping to your pizza!

- Beets: The rich red color of beets is due to high amounts of phytonutrients that the vegetable contains. Beets have high amounts of minerals and vitamins and contain the amino acid betaine. Betaine is found to help the liver function, detoxify cells from any toxins in the environment, and help cells maintain their health and normal function in the immune system. They've even been found to protect the body against heart disease and cancer, and are considered a "brain food", or a food that helps increase blood flow to the brain. Try and incorporate beets into your salads and include it in your vegetable drawer.

- Soy: Tofu, edamame, and soy milk are all great ways to absorb the healthy benefits of soy products. Isoflavones that are present in soy products can be linked to lower inflammation in patients, and women specifically. Soy also helps keep the bones and heart healthy. Try and use soy milk when making smoothies so you can enjoy the benefits of it coupled with all the other fruits and veggies you are eating.

Shopping Guide

So what tips can we give you to plan for a better diet that can hopefully reduce the symptoms of arthritis and inflammation in your life? It's important that you know what foods you should be stocking up in your pantry, and what types of food you should be avoiding altogether. Here are some tips to get you started when you're browsing the grocery store aisles!

- Fresh Fruits and Vegetables: We've seen with the many examples listed above that a wide variety of fruits and vegetables consumed allow you to intake the most vitamins and minerals in your diet. Try and find fresh produce. If you cannot afford organic produce, that's okay, but try and buy a few things organic such as leafy green vegetables like kale and spinach, or soft-flesh fruits where the skin will be eaten, like peaches and plums. Different colored fruits also have different beneficial properties, like red fruits and vegetables (apples, red bell peppers, strawberries), as well as darker skin fruits and vegetables (blackberries, eggplants, blueberries), so be sure to have a colorful array of items in your shopping cart!

- Chicken and Turkey: These poultry items are great alternatives to red meat, especially for patients who might already be battling high cholesterol or heart disease. Try and find fresh cuts and avoid processed or pre-made frozen meals that could have preservatives or high amounts of sodium.

- Fish: The benefits of omega-3 fatty acids have been praised over and over in this chapter, so we urge you to buy some fish this grocery trip! Whether it's tuna, mackerel, salmon, or tilapia, explore your options and recipes so you can incorporate fish into your meals at least twice a week.

- Olive Oil: The benefits of olive oil are like ibuprofen, but naturally! It's found to lower inflammation and reduce pain. Be sure that you have olive oil to use when cooking or as dressing on salads and pasta. Try and find brands that come with a seal of approval like the North American Olive Oil Seal. If you can splurge on extra virgin olive oil which is less refined, even better! But regular olive oil should become a staple in your pantry.

- Whole Wheat Grains and Cereals: Try and find grains that are whole wheat without any sodium or additives. Also look for cereals that are packed with iron or fiber, so you are hitting your daily intake limit without needing to take over the counter supplements.

- Yogurt and Dairy: Despite some studies that have dairy as aggravating arthritis symptoms, yogurts, milk, and cheeses provide many health benefits.

- Ginger and Garlic: As stated above, ginger and garlic are two substances that have natural ingredients that reduce inflammation in the body. Try and incorporate these two foods in your diet whether it's minced garlic on a salad or crushed ginger in soups or slaws.

- Juices: As mentioned above, many vegetable juices have been linked to decreased inflammation such as tomato juice and beet juice. It's important that these juices contain fewer sugars and additives. They should use the most organic ingredients possible. Whether you're making them at home or finding them at the grocery store, be sure that you are keeping the fruit or vegetable in as pure a state as you can.

- Teas: Herbal green tea has been found to have antioxidant and anti-inflammatory properties. A study at Washington State University found that a molecule in green tea works to target a pro-inflammatory protein that is found in high quantities in patients with rheumatoid arthritis. It is important to note that green tea contains traces of vitamin K which can counteract blood thinners. If you are on blood thinners, it's important you talk to your doctor before you incorporate green tea into your diet.

- Avoid Processed Sugary Foods: Sorry, but junk food has to stay in the store! If you are trying to maintain a healthy lifestyle and promote weight loss, stay away from processed snacks that are loaded with sugars or corn syrup. Try and find alternatives that fall under "healthy snacking" such as lentil chips or salt-free popcorn.

Chapter 7: Drinks & Smoothies That Reduce Inflammation

As discussed in the previous chapter, many foods, especially fruits and vegetables, can fight symptoms of inflammation and arthritis. It's all about adjusting your diet to a healthy one full of lots of good fats and a variety of vitamins and minerals. You also want to make sure you're avoiding trans fats, alcohol, and sugars that can cause flare-ups of inflammation. You want to increase foods in your diet that agree with your digestion and that are helpful to fight inflammation.

Smoothies are a great way to pack a lot of vitamins and minerals into just one cup. They're easy to make and easy to take on the go! Gathering the right ingredients is simple as long as you have them already stocked in your fridge and pantry. That's where the helpful shopping guide in the earlier chapter comes handy! To make it even easier on yourself amid a busy schedule, you can even portion out ingredients and keep them in freezer-safe bags so it's as easy as pouring and mixing your smoothie.

You want to pack your drinks with many of the ingredients we mentioned that can combat signs of inflammation. Here are some additions that go well in smoothies to further help you and your health.

- ✓ Turmeric: This Asian spice has become very popular in the West in recent years because of its enormous health benefits. It's known for reducing chronic inflammation in the body by blocking the chemicals that trigger inflammation to occur. Just a teaspoon of this spice is all you need to gain the benefits, and it adds a bright yellow color to your drinks! That's due to a pigment called curcumin that is found in turmeric.

✓ Ginger: This is another substance that reduces inflammation. It might not sound so tasty in a morning smoothie, but just adding a few small pieces of ginger can have a beneficial effect. Try and mix it with other strong ingredients, such as fruits that have natural sugars, or soy milk that can cover up the taste. You might have to do some experiments to find the right flavor balance, but don't leave this ingredient out!

✓ Berries: These are perfect for a smoothie and work naturally to fight inflammation in the body. Packed with natural antioxidants and tons of vitamins and minerals, there's so many for you to choose from depending on your favorite flavors! Blueberries, strawberries, raspberries... even cherries and pomegranate seeds are a great addition to any smoothie. And they're naturally sweet so you can cut back on any sugar you would have added!

✓ Chia Seeds: These little seeds have become the star in many dishes lately. Despite their size, they are packed with omega-3 fatty acids that work to combat inflammation in the body. By increasing the amount of fatty acids we eat, we can hopefully see inflammation reduce. Be sure to include a handful of these in your smoothie. They're mostly tasteless so you won't even know they're there!

✓ Greens: Spinach, kale, chard... yes, a green smoothie is synonymous with a healthy smoothie because it's the truth! They are high in antioxidants and enzymes that enter your bloodstream and break down molecules that cause inflammation. The more raw your greens are consumed, the more effective they are. Be sure to include a cup of greens in your smoothie is the best way to have your daily intake. Kale is considered a superfood because it is high in so many vitamins and minerals including riboflavin, iron, magnesium, and Vitamins A, K, B6, and C. Experiment with what combinations and amounts work best for you, and how you can combine them with a mix of other fruits and other vegetables.

√ Apples: Though apples sometimes get looked over for other sweeter fruits, red apples have been researched and found to have antioxidants in their skin that act as a natural anti-inflammatory. Studies even found that people who eat three to five apples a week have a lower risk of developing asthma, which is an inflammatory condition. You can use green apples if you prefer the tartness, but don't forget some slices of apple in your smoothie to get all the nutrients!

√ Pineapples: This delicious tropical fruit is rich in Vitamin C and an enzyme called bromelain. This enzyme digests other proteins, such as the ones that are causing trouble in the body by creating inflammation! It can reduce swelling, pain, and bruising in the body and give you arthritis and tendonitis relief. If you can find this fresh, it is a great addition to include in your smoothies - for the health benefits and the taste! If not, you can always find it canned but make sure you read the label and find the one with the least amount of artificial sugar.

√ Nuts: When making your smoothie, be sure to add in a handful of nuts. Almonds are high in unsaturated fatty acids that work to keep the joints lubricated. Walnuts also contain similar fatty acids that release acids to protect the body from bone loss. Walnuts inhibit the production of neurotransmitters that cause pain and inflammation. Be sure that you are adding raw nuts and not a salty or sugary type.

✓ Kiwi: A fruit that's not paid too much attention to, recent research has shown that kiwis are packed with antioxidants and anti-inflammatory proteins. They are rich in fiber, vitamin E, potassium, vitamin K, and so many others! They are a tart and tangy fruit so if you can't eat it raw, it's great to include in your smoothies with other ingredients to balance or hide the flavor.

Here are some great recipes to get you started on making smoothies! The great thing about smoothies is that they are so versatile and it is easy to switch ingredients. If you don't prefer blueberries, try a different berry like blackberries. If you don't care for pistachios, try walnuts instead. These recipes are for making 1 serving so if you are having guests, feel free to double it!

Greek Yogurt Smoothie: This smoothie is filled with proteins, so it's perfect as a post-workout treat when the body is looking for proteins to rebuild muscle. It's also very filling so it can even replace dinner if you are trying to lose weight and maintain a healthier lifestyle. As mentioned, feel free to use whichever berries you prefer. Also, if you have another leafy green you like better, you can switch out the spinach for kale.

.25 cup Greek yogurt, plain, no additives
1 cup nut milk, like cashew, almond, or soy
.25 cup baby spinach
.25 cup blueberries
2 tablespoons peanut butter

.25 teaspoon of cinnamon

a few ice cubes

Strawberry Red Smoothie: This smoothie is packed with sweet and tart ingredients that are packed with vitamins and minerals. The beautiful red color makes it already look delicious!

.5 cup red beets, peeled and chopped

a small half-inch piece of ginger, peeled

.75 cup cranberry juice

.75 cup strawberries

a pinch of cinnamon

1 tablespoon organic honey

a few ice cubes if you prefer!

Tropical Summer Smoothie: This smoothie is a beautiful yellow and is so delicious that you won't even remember how good it is for your health! With delicious tropical fruits, it's the best treat, especially on a hot summer day.

1 cup mango, fresh or frozen

1.5 cup cold water

a few ice cubes

1 teaspoon turmeric

a small half-inch piece of ginger, peeled

1 cup pineapple, fresh or frozen

.5 teaspoon coconut oil

Sweet Potato Smoothie: Both spinach and sweet potatoes are healthy vegetables that can reduce inflammation. They're also a great source of magnesium. A magnesium deficiency can lead to muscle cramps.

.5 cup sweet potato, cooked

.5 cup almond milk

.5 teaspoon vanilla extract

a handful of baby spinach

1 teaspoon honey

a pinch of cinnamon

a small half-inch piece of ginger, peeled

a half banana

Pineapple Turmeric Smoothie: Combined with turmeric and ginger, this fruit smoothie is a powerful tool to combat inflammation - and it's delicious! Try and find the freshest fruit you can, but if you can't, feel free to experiment with substitutes.

a small half-inch piece of ginger, peeled

1 teaspoon turmeric

.5 cup pineapple

.5 cup mango

.5 cup coconut milk

.5 teaspoon vanilla extract

a pinch of cardamom powder (or cinnamon, if you don't have it!)

Avocado Citrus Smoothie: Avocados are a superfood and contain high amounts of folic acid, vitamin C, vitamin E, and more than a dozen other nutrients! With some citrus fruit added as well, this smoothie is packed with tons of vitamin C.

1 avocado chopped into pieces

juice of 1 small orange

juice of 1 small lemon

.5 teaspoon vanilla extract

1 cup milk of your choice

1 banana

a few cubes of ice

Carrot Ginger Smoothie: Packed with tons of ingredients to combat inflammation, along with lots of Vitamin C, this smoothie is full of antioxidants and will fulfill some of your fruit and vegetable servings for the day.

.5 cup cold water

a small piece of ginger root

juice of 1 small lemon

1 teaspoon turmeric

.5 cup carrots, peeled and chopped

.5 cup pineapple, fresh or frozen

.5 cup milk of your choice

1 large ripe banana

Kiwi Ginger Smoothie: This smoothie shines on the healing power of kiwis that are believed to have anti-inflammatory proteins. It's a tangy fruit so feel free to add a handful of berries or a teaspoon of honey if you feel like you need to sweeten the flavor. Adding in nuts and gives you a boost of healthy fat and proteins too!

2 kiwis, peeled and chopped

1 ripe banana

a small piece of ginger root

4 tablespoons cashews

.5 cup water

a few ice cubes

1 teaspoon of chia seeds

Strawberry Almond Smoothie: A simple smoothie consisting of berries and almonds, this is a great way to get your daily fruit intake, and some "good" fats with a handful of nuts! Almond milk is a great milk to use because it is packed with nutrients and gives more flavor than regular milk.

.5 cup strawberries
1 cup almond milk, unsweetened
.5 cup orange juice, natural
.5 cup yogurt, no additives

Coconut and Ginger Smoothie: As we shared in the previous chapter, ginger is known for its medicinal anti-inflammatory properties. It can combat nausea, digestive issues, and believed to even stop the growth of cancer cells! This is a great and simple smoothie to have a healthy helping of ginger.

1 ripe banana
.5 cup coconut milk
a pinch of cinnamon
a pinch of nutmeg
5-10 few pieces of ginger root, about an inch each, how many depends on how strong a flavor you like

Cucumber Pineapple Smoothie: Pineapples are high in bromelain which has been studied and found to inhibit inflammation and pain. With a hint of cinnamon to regulate blood sugar, this is a great treat of flavors.

.5 cup pineapple chunks
2 small cucumbers, peeled and diced
.5 teaspoon cinnamon powder

.5 teaspoon turmeric powder

Blueberry Green Juice: This smoothie is just three ingredients but each one has unique properties to fight inflammation. Blueberries contain the most antioxidants compared to other fruits and vegetables, and spinach is high in folic acid!
1 cup blueberries, fresh or frozen
.5 cup Fuji apples, peeled and chopped
1 cup fresh spinach leaves
.5 cup cold water
a few ice cubes

Watermelon Smoothie: This smoothie is perfect as a summertime treat. Even though watermelon is made up of mostly water, it's filled with a powerful antioxidant called lycopene. Lycopene works to protect the skin and internal organs and reduces inflammation in the body by neutralizing free radical ions. Other nutrients work to block the enzyme that causes pain and inflammation in the body. Be sure to pick the ripest watermelon you can find so you get all the nutrients you can!

3 cups watermelon, skin and seeds removed, cut into chunks
7-8 small basil leaves, fresh (use less if bigger size)
juice of half a lime

Conclusion

Thank you for making it through to the end of *Arthritis Diet!* We hope that by reading this book some of your questions about arthritis and inflammation were answered. These are serious afflictions that millions of people live with on a daily basis, especially the elderly. Adjusting one's life to this disease and the constant swelling or pain accompanied with it can be devastating. Trying to maintain an active lifestyle if you had one before can become challenging. Whether you were simply looking for more information on these conditions or wondering about the causes for it, we hope this book has been informative in providing you answers. It's important to note that despite many potential causes of arthritis such as family history, lifestyle choices, and obesity, the majority of researchers believe that arthritis is a disease that the human body will eventually succumb to, no matter how healthy or active you are. That is simply how the human body is set up. Over time, the cartilage and joints begin to break down due to the body's weight and activities.

Before making any changes in your exercise or diet, you should speak to your primary care doctor regarding your arthritis pain. They may have other suggestions in mind or make you aware of any conflicts regarding medication you're taking. Making the switch to a vegan or vegetarian diet is also a big change and a doctor should be consulted.

If you're looking to make healthier choices in your diet and meals to ease arthritis symptoms and boost your immune system, we hope we've provided you with some great tips to get started. We've provided a great list of foods that you can incorporate more into your weekly menu. Foods like fish, beans, citrus fruits, and leafy green vegetables should be eaten a few times a week. Fruits and vegetables especially are very important, and if you can buy them organic, it's even better. Leafy vegetables like spinach and kale contain a variety of antioxidants that have been found to block the proteins that signal inflammation. Even adding just a little bit of minced garlic or ginger to your meals can be helpful too. And don't forget the olive oil! This oil is known to have medicine-like properties and should be used by arthritis patients in their meal preparation.

When talking about a healthier arthritis diet, it's also necessary to cut the processed, salty, or sugary snacks. It's especially important if you are trying to lose weight in order to ease your symptoms of arthritis. Excess weight puts pressure on the joints of the body and this stress speeds up the process of cartilage breaking down. Smoothies are a great way to pack many healthy ingredients into a drink, so you are getting as many nutrients as you can in the raw form. With the right ingredients, they can also be very filling and help you maintain a goal weight if you are struggling with meals. We've included nearly a dozen smoothie recipes so you can pick and choose the perfect treat for your flavor profile!

We hope that this book has given you some ideas on how to eat a healthier diet in hopes of reducing your pain and inflammation!

Plant-Based Nutrition:

Guide on How to Eat Healthy and For a Healthier Body

Introduction

Congratulations on purchasing the *Plant-Based Nutrition* and thank you for doing so.

The typical American diet is not healthy at all. Many people eat way too much processed foods and junk foods. They spend their time going out to eat, rather than making a healthy and delicious meal from home. When they do eat at home, they rarely enjoy foods that are full of nutrition and the healthy vitamins and minerals that they need. Instead, they focus on eating quick-to-make meals, ones that ruin their health despite being easier to make.

Even some popular diet plans out there—ketogenic diet, for one—can be harmful for the health. Studies have long shown that these kinds of diets, while popular, are going to cause more chronic illnesses and will lead to a shorter lifespan. What could be the solution?

A plant-based diet is the one and only plan that you need to follow to help reduce your risks of many chronic health conditions and to ensure that you have more energy and an increased lifespan. This type of eating asks you to focus on foods like legumes, whole grains, and plenty of fruits and vegetables. If you can do this, and add enough variety to your meals, you can easily get the nutrients that you need while also improving your health.

There are some variations to this kind of diet plan, though. With a vegetarian diet, you would still consume some dairy products on occasion, and some even allow fish to help get all the healthy nutrients inside. The Mediterranean diet is another plant-based diet that allows fish and a little bit of red meat, as long as it is kept to a minimum serving and is just there as a complement to the plant-based foods. Or, you can start on a vegan diet, which focuses just on eating plant-based foods. No matter which option you go with, plant-based nutrition is only going to spell out good things for your mind, body, and soul.

This guidebook spends some time talking about the health benefits of a plant-based diet and why it is so good for you. Many people are used to eating meat and sticking with the regular diet that they have always known. These same people often wonder why they are fighting diabetes, cancer, heart disease, and other chronic illnesses. With a plant-based diet, you can reduce these illnesses, and in some cases, you can even reverse them! Never disregard or forget the old saying: "Prevention is better than cure"

When you are ready to learn more about a plant-based diet, and what plant-based nutrition can do for you, look no further than this guidebook. It has all the information that you need to help you get started!

There are plenty of books on this subject on the market. Thanks again for choosing this one! Every effort was made to ensure it is full of as much useful information as possible. Please enjoy!

Chapter 1: What is Plant-Based Nutrition?

Plant-based nutrition is when an individual decides to consume a diet that is full of whole plant foods. This includes plenty of fruits, vegetables, legumes, and even whole grain products. These nutrients provide the body with everything it needs, with none of the bad stuff that our typical American diet introduces to the body. Plant-based nutrition is able to provide the body with all of the nutrients it needs, from fiber, minerals, vitamins, fat, protein, and carbs. It can even provide you with adequate calories to get through the day.

There are many reasons that an individual will choose to go on a plant-based diet. Some may do it as a lifestyle choice to help improve their health; others will pick ethical, religious, or cultural reasons to follow plant-based nutrition. This is also a great way to keep oneself healthy and to prevent a lot of health problems, including diabetes and heart disease. No matter what the reason for choosing a plant-based diet is, the benefits are truly amazing and can help you feel better than you can ever imagine.

There are decades of research that shows how most chronic health issues are directly linked back to lifestyle choices and diet. The science supports the idea of adopting a more plant-based diet to help prevent and even reverse a lot of these chronic illnesses. People who follow a diet that consists mostly of animal source foods are the ones who tend to get more of these chronic diseases. People who eat a diet that is mostly plant-based are the healthiest and often avoid these chronic diseases.

One of these studies that really support this claim is known as "The China Study". This was done by Dr. T. Colin Campbell and it's one of the most comprehensive long-term studies on nutrition. It focused on the relationship between the diet the individuals followed and their risks of developing a disease. The findings ended up challenging much of what the typical American diet believes.

In this study, it was found that those populations that consumed high carbohydrates were trimmer, healthier, and more vibrant compared to others. The diet of those found in this study consisted mostly of rice, vegetables, a little fish, and no dairy products at all. The Okinawans, the group that was studied, have more people living over 100 years old per 100,000 in population than anywhere else in the world. And they also have the lowest death rates from stroke, heart disease, and cancer, with the highest life expectancy for everyone.

That is just one example of how a plant-based diet can really help you to improve your health. Individuals who focus more on eating healthy legumes, whole grains, and fresh produce, tend to live longer and have fewer chronic illnesses compared to others. Especially when compared to the typical diet found in the Western world right now.

Another example of this is Asia where healthy people there thrive on high-carbohydrate, rice-based diets. The Japanese, who stick with a pretty traditional diet, eat plenty of vegetables and rice with just small amounts of animal protein. The people of this country tend to have lower incidents of prostate, colon, and breast cancer, fewer incidents of heart disease, and have the best longevity out of the world.

Or, you can look at the Seventh-Day Adventists. They adhere to a strict vegetarian diet, which follows plant-based nutrition. They stick with mostly vegetables, fruits, legumes, and grains in order to follow their religion. These individuals also tend to have a lower incident of colon cancer and heart disease when compared to others in the same country.

The goal of the plant-based diet is to fill the body with exactly the types of nutrients that it needs to thrive and do well. Focus on eating foods that are whole and delicious, ones that will fill you up and give you the energy and the nutrients that are needed to fight off many illnesses that are common today. Simply by sticking with fruits, vegetables, legumes, and whole grains, you can give your body exactly what it needs to be healthy.

Is Plant-Based Nutrition Complicated to Follow?

Getting started with plant-based nutrition is not that difficult. In fact, you will be surprised at how easy it can be. And, depending on your level of comfort, you can even make some changes to have it work better for you. Each person follows a plant-based diet in a different manner, and some people may be on this kind of eating plan without even really noticing.

To be on a true plant-based diet, you need to cut out all the animal products. This includes milk, eggs, and all the meats including beef, fish, pork, bacon, chicken, veal, and more. This allows you to focus on eating whole and fresh ingredients, like fresh produce, whole grains, and legumes. There are also some substitutes, such as almond milk and other non-dairy milk that can be used if this is hard to stick with. You'll be surprised to find that there are a lot of substitutes in the market today on just about any food item. You just have to be patient, and do some research. You need to invest your time and effort for a much healthier lifestyle. As long as you're determined to do so, anything is possible.

But, modifications are allowed in some cases. For example, some people choose to follow a vegetarian diet that allows some fish. Those who follow the Mediterranean diet–a form of the plant-based diet–find that they can have a bit of red meat once or twice a month, and some fish; but they mostly need to follow the rules of the plant-based diet. Or, you can choose to do the vegan version of this diet plan, which simply has to stick with the three main food groups that we have discussed.

That is the beauty of this eating plan. You get to choose how you follow it. As long as the primary source of your nutrition comes from the whole grains, legumes, and fresh produce, you can have some freedom on the diet you choose. Eating in this way is going to make such a difference in your whole life and it can make you feel healthier and happier in no time. It may seem difficult in the beginning, but give it just a few weeks and you are sure to see the benefits and you will find that this is not as difficult as you have thought.

Chapter 2: The Health Benefits of Plant-Based Nutrition

There are a lot of health benefits that come with following a plant-based nutrition program. This diet may be different from what you are used to with your traditional diet, but the benefits are amazing and you only need to make a few tweaks in the way that you eat right now. Here, we are going to explore some of the health benefits that come with following a plant-based diet and why it is something you should consider doing today!

Prevents Chronic Diseases

Everyone has heard the saying "An apple a day keeps the doctor away." and it seems that this piece of advice may be true. A diet that is high in vegetables and fruits can help prevent many chronic illnesses. There are numerous studies out there that show how a plant-based diet can protect you against diabetes and cancer.

Why does this happen? A plant-based diet is naturally low in saturated fats, low in added sugar, and high in fiber, compared to processed foods or animal-based foods. This means that when you go on this kind of diet, you can lower your blood pressure, improve your levels of blood sugar, and lose weight.

Even if you start out small, you are going to see some big changes. In a 2016 study published by PLOS Medicine, it was discovered that even little tweaks in your diet can really lower your risk of diabetes. Simply cutting your daily servings of animal products from six to four could help. And, if you adhere to the ideas of a plant-based diet, you could even reverse diabetes in those who already have the disease.

Gets Rid of the Brain Fog

Many people who decide to go on a plant-based diet are impressed by how much easier it is for them to focus and concentrate on the task at hand. It may be because you are helping to provide the mind with the nutrients it needs to function properly. It may only take a few days of being on this type of eating plan to see the benefits and to be amazed at how quickly you can get the work done as compared to before.

Improves Your Mood

Beyond being able to reduce your risk of many common illnesses such as diabetes and cancer, eating a diet that has tons of fresh produce can actually increase how happy you feel. So, while eating berries and lots of fresh produce is good for your physical health when you add it as part of your lifestyle, it can also be good when it comes to your mental health.

A recent study that was done in 2016 and published in the American Journal of Public Health found that by increasing your consumption of fresh produce over a two-year period is equal to the size of the psychological gain of moving from unemployment to employment.

What is the reason for this? One possible reason is that a plant-based diet is able to provide your body with the antioxidants it needs to fight inflammation and the phytochemicals that can help regulate the brain chemicals that control your mood. This results in you feeling happier more often.

Protects Your Heart

You can use the idea of plant-based nutrition in order to help your heart get stronger than ever before. With lots of whole grains, vegetables, and fruits, you can make sure that the heart is strong and is getting all the nutrients it needs. With all these healthy foods, you can help lower your blood pressure, which can do wonders for the strength and health of your heart. Studies have shown that vegetarianism can help you reduce your risk of heart disease by at least 33%!

It goes even further than that. It is believed that a diet full of greens and fresh produce may be able to turn off the genes that make individuals more susceptible to heart disease. This is the power of plants. Known as epigenetics, or the science of how your lifestyle can interact with your genes, these studies have found that certain genetic variations that can increase your risk of heart disease can be countered when you make certain changes in your lifestyle, such as adopting a plant-based diet.

Keeps off the Excess Weight

Many people who choose to go on one of the plant-based diets do it in order to help them keep off the extra weight. When it comes to gimmicky diets and calorie counting, no one wants to spend their time worrying about these. This can be discouraging and really hard to do on a regular basis.

When you go on a plant-based diet, you can avoid all of these. There are no tricks to this kind of diet plan. Just make sure that you pick fresh legumes, whole grains, and fresh produce. Then, in addition to helping with the above mood and health benefits, you can lose weight at the same time!

A study that was published in the Journal of the Academy of Nutrition and Dietetics looked at fifteen of the most common plant-based diets. They found that on average, participants were about to drop about 7.48 pounds. This includes those who didn't stick with the diet for the long term. The fiber content in this diet can sometimes lead you to feel satisfied easier, which can help with weight loss.

Adds More Energy and Longevity

Those who decide that a plant-based diet is the right option for them may find that they can live longer. Studies show that a vegetarian diet and other plant-based diets are associated with a lower risk of death. And if you follow the Mediterranean diet, which is another plant-based diet that is popular and has amazing health benefits, you will have a longer telomere length, which basically translates into better health and longevity.

Basically, it doesn't matter which of the plant-based diets you choose to follow. All of them can be beneficial to your health. And if you follow them well and for a long time, they could help you to increase your energy and can help you increase your longevity all at the same time.

These are just a few of the great health benefits you will be able to get when you decide to go on a plant-based diet. There are tons of great recipes and resources that you can use–including what we provide in this guidebook–to help you get started on this type of eating plan. It is easy, it is healthy, and it can help you live a much better life than before!

Chapter 3: Breakdown of Plant Vitamins and Minerals

Many people worry that if they do decide to go on a plant-based diet, they won't be able to provide their bodies with the right nutrients. They see that they should eliminate dairy food products and wonder how they will get their daily calcium. They see that they need to kick out animal source foods, like beef and chicken, and wonder how they will get some important nutrients like protein and the B vitamins. A plant-based diet is actually a great way to ensure you get plenty of vitamins and minerals. And, compared to the highly processed diet you ate before, you will end up getting way more of these important nutrients into your diet than you did before.

For those who are concerned about getting enough of specific nutrients in your daily diet when you follow plant-based nutrition, it is useful to know what kinds of foods that contain each type of nutrient. This helps you to add enough variety into your meal to actually get the nutrients that the body needs. And if you find that you have fallen behind on some of your daily recommendations, you can always throw together a few fruits and vegetables and make a smoothie to finish out your day.

Let's take a look at where you can find these nutrients in a plant-based diet plan:

- Calcium: You can find calcium in a wide variety of places. These include dried fruits, dried figs, Brazil nuts, flaxseeds, almonds, sunflower seeds, sesame seeds, most beans, chickpeas, blackstrap molasses, tofu, and green leafy vegetables such as kale, spinach, and broccoli. You can easily get plenty of calcium in your day without having to rely on dairy milk.

- Iron: Again, the green leafy vegetables, as well as sea vegetables, can help with this. Other options include whole grains, cereals, prune juice, watermelon, dried fruits, blackstrap molasses, nuts and seeds, legumes, and beans.

- Magnesium: This nutrient is found in options like peanuts, bananas, green leafy vegetables, whole grains, wheat germ or bran, cooked oatmeal, dried figs, almonds and nuts, beans and legumes, cooked spinach, and brown rice.

- Phosphorus: You can find this nutrient in options like yeast, spinach, avocados, brown rice, peanuts, lentils, peas, dried beans, nuts, almonds, cereal grains, and pinto beans.

- Potassium: This nutrient can be found in options like dried apricots, cantaloupe, melon, strawberries, kiwifruit, winter squash, baked potatoes, cooked spinach, raisins, and bananas.

- Zinc: This nutrient can be found in sources like corn, spinach, raw collard greens, garbanzo beans, yeast, wheat germ, sunflower seeds, nuts, soy foods, peas, lentils, legumes, cereals and whole grains, and pumpkin seeds.

- Selenium: You can find this nutrient in many places including mustard seeds, asparagus, seeds, tofu, whole grains, mushrooms, and Brazil nuts.
- Manganese: You can find this nutrient in some options like strawberries, pineapples, avocados, almonds, black beans,

kale, spinach, legumes, seeds, wheat germ, nuts, cooked oatmeal, cereals, whole grains, and brown rice.

- Biotin: You can find this nutrient in options like legumes, molasses, peanuts, almonds, yeast, bread, whole grains, and cereals.

- Folic Acid: This nutrient is very important when it comes to being pregnant, or when you are trying to get pregnant. Some of the sources of this nutrient include romaine lettuce, spinach, asparagus, whole grains, oranges, lentils, and legumes.

- Vitamin B1 or Thiamine: Even though many people worry that a plant-based diet will leave them without any of the B vitamins, you will soon see this is not true. You can get this nutrient from raw wheat germs, watermelon, nuts, sunflower seeds, cereals, legumes, nutritional yeast, oatmeal, pasta, bread, whole grains, and brown rice.

- Niacin or Vitamin B3: You can get this from tomatoes, potatoes, green vegetables, brown rice, and legumes.

- Vitamin B6: You can get this nutrient from whole grains, watermelon, bananas, walnuts, soybeans, nuts, and legumes.

- Vitamin B12: This one is a bit harder to get, but there are some cereals and non-dairy milk that are fortified with this nutrient.

- Vitamin C: This nutrient is best for keeping you healthy, especially during the winter. Some of the places you can get this nutrient from includes watercress, romaine lettuce, papayas, berries, melon, potatoes, spinach, collard greens, tomatoes, grapefruit, oranges and orange juice, strawberries, tomatoes, broccoli, and bell peppers.

- Vitamin D: You can get exposure to this just by being out in the sun, no matter which diet plan you are on. You can also find it in some cereals and milk.

- Vitamin E: You can get this from whole grains, spinach, green leafy vegetables, sunflower seeds, and vegetable oils.

- Pantothenic acid: You can find this nutrient in options like broccoli, baked potato, collard greens, oranges, bananas, sunflower seeds, avocados, soybeans, peanuts, mushrooms, legumes, and whole grain cereals.

- Vitamin K: This would include options like tomatoes, green tea, cabbage, broccoli, parsley, kale, turnip greens, spinach, soybean oil, and green leafy vegetables.

As you look through this list, you should notice that all of these are options that are based on a plant-based diet plan. And there are so many more nutrients that you would be able to get from these as well. But for many individuals who are worried about going on a plant-based diet because they think they will miss out on all of the nutrients that their body needs, just look at this list. You simply need to go through and check that your meals have a lot of variety in them so you can reach all those nutrient goals.

Chapter 4: Checklist of What to Eat and What Not to Eat

When you are ready to start a plant-based diet, one question that you may have is what is safe to eat and what you need to avoid. There are so many different diet plans out there, and, sometimes, things can get confusing. You want to make sure that you eat the right kinds of foods and avoid the wrong ones so you can get the full benefits of a plant-based diet.

The plant-based diet focuses primarily on foods that come from plants. The thought here is that these plant foods have tons of nutrients, the nutrients that the body is craving without having any of the bad stuff in them. If you can stick with a diet that is full of these plants, you are going to be able to keep your health nice and strong. Let's take a look at some of the different types of foods you can eat on a plant-based diet.

Foods to Eat on a Plant-Based Diet

The first area we are going to look at is some of the foods that you should focus on when you go with a plant-based diet. These are pretty simple to stick with, and there is a lot of variety so you should never get bored. Some of the different food groups you will focus on here include:

- Fruits: Get a wide variety of fruits into this diet. In fact, fill up your plate during every meal! Some good options here include bananas, pineapple, peaches, pears, mangoes, papayas, oranges, and berries.

- Vegetables: Vegetables are a great source of nutrition and you would be surprised at how far a little bit can go. Some of the vegetables that you should enjoy on a plant-based diet include bell peppers, asparagus, carrots, cauliflower, broccoli, tomatoes, spinach, and kale.

- Whole grains: Grains are great for this diet as long as you make sure you pick the whole grain variety. Go with options like barley, oats, quinoa, hemp, farro, and brown rice.

- Healthy fats: Fats are allowed on this diet plan. Some of the best options for this food group include unsweetened coconut, coconut oil, olive oil, and avocados.

- Legumes: This would include anything that falls into the category of black beans, peanuts, lentils, chickpeas, and peas.

- Nut butters, nuts, and seeds: There are a lot of great options that work here including tahini, peanut butter, sunflower seeds, pumpkin seeds, macadamia nuts, cashews, and almonds.

- Unsweetened and plant-based milk: Go with options like cashew milk, almond milk, soya milk, oat milk, and coconut milk.

- Seasonings, herbs, and spices: These are just fine to add to your diet and can be a much healthier option compared to using salt. Stick with options like pepper, curry, turmeric, thyme, rosemary, dill, and basil.

- Condiments: You need to be careful about some of the condiments that you have on the plant-based diet, but not all of them are bad. Some good options include lemon juice, vinegar (apple cider, balsamic, rice), soy sauce, nutritional yeast, mustard, and salsa.

- Plant-based protein: While you are on the plant-based diet, you still need to get protein to keep the body strong. The good news is you can still rely on some plant-based products to help you get that protein. Options like protein powders that don't have artificial ingredients or added sugars, tempeh, and tofu can all work well.

- Beverages: Options like sparkling water, tea, water, and coffee are just fine.

There are some people who will leave their diet right there. They just want to stick with the plant-based diet and do nothing else for that time. But others may find that it is too restrictive; or maybe they have a condition such as pregnancy, which requires them to get some animal-based products like milk and they need to be able to supplement them into the plant-based diet.

If you decide to supplement your plant-based diet with some animal products, make sure to use them only as a compliment—the plant-based foods should be the main priority here—and pick out high-quality options. Some of the options you can supplement in here include:

- Dairy: It is fine to add in dairy products on occasion. We did talk about a few plant-based options, but you can choose to add in regular dairy products on occasion if you choose. If possible, go with dairy products that are organic and from pasture-raised animals.

- Seafood: Seafood is the most common animal-based product that is added to this kind of eating. The benefits that come from fish far outweigh the negatives of eating it. Go with wild-caught fish when you can.

- Pork and beef: Go with grass-fed or pastured any time that you can.

- Poultry: Organic and free-range are the best options when possible.

- Eggs: Pasture-raised when possible.

Foods to Avoid on a Plant-Based Diet

There are also some foods you should avoid when following a plant-based diet. Some of these include:

- Any type of fast food: This would include chicken nuggets, hot dogs and sausages, pizzas, cheeseburgers, and French fries.

- Added sugars and sweets: This would include sugary cereals, sweet teas, candies, cookies, ice cream, pastries, juices, sodas, and table sugar.

- Refined grains: This would be options like white bread, bagels, white pasta, and white rice. Make sure that you consume the whole grain versions of these to stay on your plant-based diet.

- Packaged foods and other convenience foods: This would include things like frozen dinners, instant noodles, cereal bars, crackers, and chips.
- Vegan-friendly foods that are processed: These may sound healthy, but they have a lot of things in them that can be bad for you. Some examples are faux cheeses, vegan butters, and Tofurkey.

- Artificial sweeteners: Avoid options like Sweet'N Low, Splenda, and Equal.

- Processed animal products: This would include beef jerkies, corned beef, canned tunas, and other fishes, sausages, luncheon meats, and bacon.

These are foods that are commonly found in the traditional American diet that are completely unhealthy for the body and are often the cause of many chronic illnesses. While some people will supplement in a bit of chicken or fish on occasion to this diet plan, the above foods are really hard to justify because they offer a lot of health risks and no benefit at all. If you do consume any of these on your plant-based diet, do so very sparingly. But, it is still best to avoid them as much as possible.

This means that you need to be careful about the sugars and sweets that you eat as well. Having these on occasion won't technically go against the diet because they aren't animal-based products, but they still aren't the best for your health. Try to stick with healthy and wholesome foods like the fruits, vegetables, legumes, and whole wheat that we have been talking about.

Also, you may notice that we discussed not eating grains at this point, but had said that grains were fine in the previous section. The reason for this is the type of grains. The refined grains are the white bread and pasta. These look and even taste similar to what we find with the whole grain types, but they have a lot of sugars and other artificial ingredients that are not healthy for you. When choosing grains to consume, make sure you stick with whole grains, ones that have all the good nutrients and none of the bad stuff in them.

Foods That You Should Minimize

For the most part, you will want to eliminate any foods that are not listed in our first section, or which don't fall into the category of vegetable, legumes, fruits, or whole grains. Those major food groups can easily provide your body with the nutrition it needs without all of the bad stuff that can make you sick and cause chronic illnesses.

Most people on a plant-based diet will completely avoid meat, egg, and dairy products while they are on it. However, it is fine to have it on occasion if you are careful not to take in so much that it minimizes all the good that the plant-based foods provide. For example, you could have a little bit of beef at the end of the week, or a glass of milk with your supper if you choose, but minimize it as much as possible. Some of the animal source foods that you can enjoy on a very rare basis on the plant-based diet include:

- Seafood
- Dairy
- Eggs

- Poultry
- Game Meats
- Sheep
- Pork
- Beef

On one note, there are those who follow a plant-based diet who decide to eat a little fish on occasion. This is common with many cultures that rely on a plant-based diet—like the Japanese—because of all the health benefits that come from eating fish. Just make sure that when you add this to your meals, you keep it to a minimum amount of serving. Only eat this as a treat or as a complement to all the plant-based foods you should be getting in your diet.

Chapter 5: How to Begin Plant-Based Eating Habits

Now that we have taken a look at some of the different parts that come with plant-based eating, you may be wondering where, to begin with? There is so much information about the great health benefits of following this diet plan and how it can really make your life better that you want to know how to get started right away. Each person is going to follow this plan a bit differently, and their journey will be different. But if you follow the steps that we have listed here, you will be able to see success in no time!

Learn What to Eat and What to Avoid

The first step with plant-based nutrition is to learn what you are allowed to eat, and what you need to avoid. We have discussed this a bit in this guidebook earlier, but basically, you are going to reduce and eventually cut out all the animal-based products that you eat now. Some variations allow for small amounts of fish or red meat on occasion, but you want to focus more on plant-based products.

These plant-based products include options like fruits and vegetables, whole grains, and legumes. These can easily provide you with all of the health benefits that you need to live a long and healthy life. If you add in enough variety to the meal, you are going to find that you are living your best life ever when you follow plant-based nutrition.

How to Do It

There is a lot to learn about healthy eating, especially if you have been eating the traditional American diet. Before you transition, you may want to have a few days to splurge, a few days that let you say goodbye to all of those animal-based products. Some people decide to spend that time eating steaks, burgers, casseroles, pizzas, and more to enjoy them for the last time.

Then, have a start day and decide to begin. Some people gently bring themselves into the diet. They will get rid of one thing at a time until they are fully on the new diet plan. This is sometimes easier on your system, but it also leaves a lot of room for you to fall back on your old habits and not change. But when you just jump into it at once, it can be hard, but you will adjust faster and see the results in your health —and perhaps, your waistline, faster.

Make Sure to Read the Label

Never just purchase something and assume it is safe for your eating program. The best way—and really the only way—to know what is in the foods you want to eat is to read the label. Even better, avoid products that have a label to start with because this is a great way to ensure that you are sticking with unprocessed and whole foods.

Of course, there are times when processed foods are going to make it into your meals, and this is sometimes unavoidable. But it is a bad thing if you just grab something off the shelves at the grocery store without even reading it, and then add in the processed foods that way. Read through the ingredient list on everything that you purchase. If you see an ingredient and you don't know what it is, then you may want to rethink of eating it.

There are a lot of problems that come with eating processed foods. To start, these processed foods are going to be full of mystery ingredients. These ingredients can often cause issues to your health, add in a lot of toxins to the body, and are just best left alone.

One thing to note, some people who begin this diet decide to go with cheese and meat substitutes. These are not that great for optimal health. But they can be a good thing if you are using them as a transition to move over to a plant-based diet. When you pick these items, it is still best to read the label and see what ingredients are inside.

Buy Your Supplies

You may also want to consider getting a few supplies to help you get ready for plant-based diet plans. You may need to invest in some new knives to help you slice and dice all that fresh produce you are going to rely on now. You might want to get some storage containers, especially if you plan to do some freezer meals and meal planning along the way. And you can even consider getting some spices to have around for cooking.

Keep in mind that the first few shopping trips you go on with the plant-based diet could be rocky. You should leave plenty of time to shop and should consider not bringing the kids along because they can make it more difficult. Then, when you go, make sure you have a meal plan in place and a list to follow. Don't stray from that list and you are sure to have the start of plant-based nutrition in your own home.

Try out Some Meal Planning

The plant-based diet is not difficult to follow, but it will require a bit different approach to cooking than what you did before. Working with the process of meal planning can make this a bit easier to handle. You can go through and decide on what meals you want to make, what ingredients are inside, and then plan out the meals that you are going to eat for each week. Some people are ambitious and make freezer meals for the whole month at once.

A meal plan makes your life easier. You won't have to sit at the store and hope that you are picking out meals that fit into your new diet plan. It helps you to know that you are picking meals with the right nutrition. And if you add in some freezer meal preparation to the mix, you can have delicious meals ready throughout the week without having to cook when you are busy.

Pick out How Strict You Are Going to be

When you get started, you will need to take the time to pick out how strict you want to be with this plan. Some people go all-in and decide that they will only eat foods that are plant-based. Others may make some changes to help them with their daily lives. For example: if you are allergic to nuts, you may find that some of the nutrients are a little harder to get on occasion so you may decide to add in some fish or the occasional red meat to ensure that you can still get the right nutrients.

The way that you change up the program is going to depend on what best works for you. Some people follow a plant-based diet with some fish added in; while some people decide that they want to add in some milk, but can't stand any of the nut milk so they add in one cup of milk with their supper. You can make some variations if you choose. But remember that the majority of each meal needs to be plant-based, and any additions need to just be sides or complementary to this.

Find a Friend to Do It With You

Sometimes, doing things on your own can be tough. You have the best intentions, but sometimes it is hard to watch other people get to eat animal products because it makes you realize how deprived you are–or, that is how it will feel at the time. Finding someone who can do this program with you, whether they are a friend, a spouse, a family member, or someone else, can often make a big difference in how successful you can be. Anyone can do the program with you. You can help each other not feel so isolated, you can support each other, and you can hold each other accountable along the way.

Start Out Slowly

While plant-based nutrition is a great way for you to instantly improve your health and even lose weight, it can be hard to imagine life without meat or dairy products. If you ate large amounts of animal products before, going cold turkey to fit with this program is going to be really hard.

That is why it's often best to ease yourself right into it. If you are an all-or-nothing type of person, then go ahead and give it all up at once and get started. But for the rest of us, it is fine to go slowly. Maybe spend a week cutting out the dairy that you drink and eat. Then cut down to just one or two times a week having beef or chicken or another animal meat source for dinner. You can slowly go through this until you have gotten yourself on the plant-based diet, or at least as far into it as you wish to go.

Beginning your plant-based eating habits is not supposed to be difficult. There may be some time when you first start where picking out meals is hard because you aren't sure what to make or you miss taking those animal-based products. But if you can stick with these helpful hints above, you can easily get on the plant-based diet and see some results.

Chapter 6: 3 Healthy Approaches to Help You Live Longer

The nice thing about choosing a plant-based diet is that it provides you with a lot of options. There isn't one right way to follow this diet plan; you just need to go with the one that works best for you. Some people like to start out making sure they eat meals that are high quality and nutritious. Some people decide to do fasting to help repair and speed up their metabolism. Others like to take a more relaxed approach, one that allows them to slow down and not feel stressed out as much. No matter which approach you go with, it can be so good for your overall health!

Quality Meals

Quality meals are very important when you go on a plant-based diet. Since you are cutting out a few food groups including meat and dairy—you can have this on occasion but is often reduced or eliminated—you need to make sure that the other meals you consume during the day have the right amount of nutrients to keep you healthy.

Quality meals that have a lot of varieties can really help you get these done. They ensure that you are getting enough variety into your meals and that you can really get the nutrients that the body needs. An example of the kind of meals that you would enjoy with this approach includes the following meal plan:

Day 1:
- Breakfast: Oatmeal made with coconut milk and then topped with walnuts, coconut, and berries

- Lunch: You can have a large salad topped with fresh vegetables, chickpeas, pumpkin seeds, goat cheese, and avocado
- Dinner: Have butternut squash curry

Day 2:
- Breakfast: Have some full-fat plain yogurt that is topped with pumpkin seeds, unsweetened coconut, and sliced strawberries
- Lunch: Make some chili but just hold the meat
- Dinner: Some sweet potato and black bean tacos

Day 3:
- Breakfast: Have a smoothie that is made with plant-based protein powder, peanut butter, berries, and unsweetened coconut milk
- Lunch: A hummus and veggie wrap
- Dinner: Some zucchini noodles tossed with pesto and chicken meatballs

As you can see from these examples, coming up with quality meals that fit the plant-based diet isn't too difficult, and they can be delicious too. This one shows an example where some poultry was added as well. You can choose if you would like to add in the poultry or leave it out depending on how you want to do the plant-based diet.

In addition to making sure your meals are filled with lots of nutrients and lots of varieties, you can do a few other things to make sure your meals are of good quality. First, consider making more of the meals at home. This is the best way to ensure that your foods are high quality and that no artificial ingredients are added in. The foods that you make at home are often healthier and tastier than you can get at the store, even if they do take a bit longer to finish.

When it is time to eat, make sure you sit down with your family to enjoy the meal. Family time is very important and can be a great addition to your plant-based diet. Spend time talking with one another, ask each other questions, and enjoy all the nutrition and goodness that comes with the foods you enjoy together.

Fasting (Eat-Stop-Eat)

Fasting, especially intermittent fasting has become a very popular method to help people lose weight. It allows you to eat normally during most of the week, but then you add short fasts in between. Most of these fasts last less than 24 hours total.

With the Eat-Stop-Eat method, you will choose two days, non-consecutive, out of the week that you are going to fast. You will go for 24 hours without eating, instead focusing on other things during that time period. One common method to do this is that once you finish supper for the night, you don't eat anything else until supper the next day. This helps you to go the full 24 hours but doesn't have you going to bed hungry at night, which can keep some people awake.

When you do eat after your fasting period, you focus on eating healthy and wholesome plant-based foods. This helps you to maintain your energy for those fasts and can give your body the right nutrients, even when you are not eating all of the time.

If you do this fast right, you will take in fewer calories throughout the week because you go a few days without eating. That is, unless you really binge during your eating times. Eat a normal diet when necessary and this can really turn the plant-based diet into a good weight loss option as well.

When you work with the Eat-Stop-Eat method of fasting, make sure that you don't pick out two consecutive days to fast. This means don't fast on Monday and Tuesday. Instead, you can fast on Monday and Wednesday, or on Monday and Thursday. You should also pick out a day when you are going to be pretty busy anyway. This helps you because you will be so busy with work and other obligations that you won't notice the missed meals as much.

There are other types of fasting that you can consider as well. Some people like to follow the 16:8 diet where they fast for 16 hours of the day and then eat for the other 8. This has variations that you can fit to your needs. You can do longer fasts or shorter ones. The point here is to help your body reset and get back on its natural rhythm without a lot of interventions.

Rest (Flexible Fun Exercise and Sleep)

For some people, being on a strict diet plan can be tough. They get stressed out. They worry. They ultimately give up before they even get started. For these people, it is best for them to choose a more resting approach to the plant-based diet.

Our modern world is stressful enough. Trying to keep up with work, school, the kids, and all of our other obligations can be tough. Sometimes, we need to make our eating plan to be simple, something that is easier for us to follow. With this approach, we don't just eat whatever we want and hope it works. We need to learn how to relax and not be so stressed out in the day-to-day things that you try to do.

First, this approach is going to have some flexible exercise. It is a good idea to get up and do some workouts and get your body moving. Sitting around all the time can be bad for your health and your body wants to move. But we are not going to focus on 2-hour workouts each day or intense workouts that make us want to give up. You choose the type of workout and the intensity that you like and go on from there. If you miss a workout day, get outside and go for a walk with your family. Do the fitness that feels right for you.

The next aspect is to get enough sleep. How many mornings do you wake up completely exhausted? You may need some more sleep. Lack of sleep can really mess with our bodies and will make us crave lots of comfort foods to make us feel better. And, eating a lot of these comfort foods–many of which are not recommended for the plant-based diet–can add on the calories and the weight, causing a lot of health problems.

It is important that if you go with this approach, you make sure that you get plenty of rest and sleep. Set an alarm at night and when it goes off, turn everything else off, begin your bedtime routine, and then go to bed. No fighting it, no giving excuses, and no trying to get out of it. It will be the best experience that you can imagine. Make sure that your new bedtime works so you get at least eight hours of uninterrupted sleep each day.

Life is not about running around, trying to impress others, and always feeling like you are on empty. If you need to set an early bedtime to get more sleep, then do it. If you function better with a little nap, then turn out the lights and fall asleep for a few minutes.

Your health is much more important and getting enough sleep can really help.

And finally, you should have some flexibility to have fun. It is too easy to get caught up in our work and our responsibilities, but these add a lot of stress to our lives. And who wants to spend life feeling stressed out and not having any fun? You should try to add a bit of fun each day. Turn on a funny show, go out with friends, explore something new, or even sing really loud in the car at the end of the day.

All of these approaches can be great options to help you on the plant-based diet. They will help you to really focus on your health and get the right nutrients into the body, without making you stress out about a really rigorous diet plan. Choose the one that works the best for your needs, works for your lifestyle, or just seems the best for you.

Chapter 7: Shopping Guide

Following a plant-based diet doesn't need to be difficult. In fact, you can cut out several food groups from your shopping list, which means it may be possible to shorten some of your time at the grocery store. Just remember that it is best if you can keep your foods fresh and organic, if possible, and add in as much variety as possible to get more nutrients.

Why Organic and GMO-Free are the Best

When you decide to eat organic foods, you are making a choice to eat foods that haven't been treated with fungicides, herbicides, and pesticides, and the like. It is also going to support agricultural practices that will preserve and work to better the condition of the soil the food is grown on. Soil that is considered organic is going to have more nutrients, especially minerals. This can help the food taste better, while also being better for you. There are different standards of organic food that you can choose including:

- 100% organic: This means that foods contain ingredients that are organic. These foods need to be produced without any growth hormones, genetic engineering, antibiotics, pesticides, or synthetic fertilizers. These products contain a USDA seal.

- Organic: These are products that are made with a minimum of 95% organic ingredients, but the remaining 5% needs to be approved through the USDA. No ionizing radiation is allowed.

- Made with organic ingredients: For this one, you need to have a minimum of 70% organic ingredients. The right ingredients need to be agricultural products that are produced using the organic standards. These products can't have the USDA organic seal on them.

In some cases, local farms in your area may adhere to all the regulations for organic produce, but they can't afford the official certification. You can talk to the farmers directly to find out whether they follow the sustainable farming practices. Just because they don't have the seal doesn't mean they aren't organic, so just ask.

Along with this same line, a GMO is a genetically modified organism. Most of the foods that aren't organic have these GMOs on them. They are found in canola, corn, soy, and oil products that you heat. As someone who is following a plant-based diet, you need to watch out for these.

One of the best ways to avoid these GMOs is to stick with the organic foods above. This may not always work depending on where you live, the time of year, and so on, but many times you can find organic and sustainable products to eat during the day.

There are a lot of scientific claims out there talking about GMOs and whether or not they are beneficial to us. The initial theory with these GMOs was that they would help give the world new types of foods, help the environment, improve the livelihoods of those who live in rural areas, and more. But instead, these GMOs have done more harm than good, which is why a lot of people have decided to consume foods that don't contain these in them.

You have a choice when you go to the store and purchase food. It is best to go with foods that don't have GMOs in them. This helps to keep the environment and the land safe, and it ensures that you are eating the best foods for your overall health.

Where to Shop in the Store

When you walk into the store for the first time on a plant-based diet, you may be curious where you should head first. If you really like to include animal products in your diet before, you may find that some of your old favorite spots are no longer allowed. But there are still plenty of options that will help you stay healthy and following a plant-based diet.

First, focus on the fruits and vegetables. You want to get as many of these into your diet plan as possible because they are the ones that have quite a bit of nutrition. Find the fresh produce section in your grocery store and fill up your cart! Go for a lot of varieties. You want every meal to be a rainbow of colors as much as possible. This ensures that you get a lot of varieties that will prevent boredom and helps you get plenty of nutrition.

Next, you can move on to the beans. This section is going to be in different places depending on your grocery store. Stay away from the canned variety if you can help it. These often add a lot of salt and other bad stuff into the diet that can be harmful to your health. Dry beans are the best and only take a little bit more work.

Next are the whole grains. Any grain product is fine, as long as it is in the whole grain family. Bread and pasta work nicely here and can really help to complete your meal. Sometimes, these are close together; sometimes, they are further apart so you may have to visit different places to find them. If you can, consider getting some bread or other whole grain products straight from the bakery. These taste so much better and can add some good variety to your meals.

The other parts of the store you visit will depend on what version of this you are going with. For example, if you decide to add in some fish, then go ahead and visit this part of the store. If you decide to have some dairy products, then you need to visit this part of the store as well. You can also find some non-dairy options for milk as well, so consider whether you need those as well.

Rather than wandering around the store and having to go back and forth as you remember things, go into your grocery store armed with a shopping list. Preplan your meals ahead of time so you know the exact ingredients that you need to get while you are there. This can help you to make informed decisions and can keep you on track when you are tempted.

Make sure to stay away from the center aisles of the store. This is where the sweet and snack foods are located in the store. You need to limit the amounts of sweets and snacks that you have in this diet plan. You also need to stay away from the dairy section, unless you chose to add that in, and the meat section since you will get your protein from other sources.

Why You Should Avoid the Freezer Section

Even if a product says it is vegetarian-friendly or vegan-friendly, if it is in the freezer section, you should probably stay away from it. If you need to get some frozen fruits and vegetables out of that section because your options for fresh produce are minimal that time of the year, that is fine. Just make sure to check the label to see if any bad stuff has been added. But when it comes to other foods in the freezer section, such as instant meals, frozen meals, and microwave meals, just skip this section altogether.

Many American families love the freezer section. This is the first one they head to when they get to the grocery store. It is full of meals that are quick and easy to make, which can help take the stress off during the week when you are busy. The problem is that none of these meals are healthy for you at all.

Take a look at the ingredients on the box of some of your favorite frozen meals. Are you able to pronounce half of them? If you are like most people, you just grab the box and leave. But if you would look at the label, you would be surprised at what is in your food.

Even in options that are supposed to be healthy for you and are supposed to be vegan-friendly and vegetarian-friendly, you may find that the labels tell a different story. Some may even have animal products in them, like eggs and milk. Add in all the preservatives, the artificial ingredients, the sodium, and other harmful additions; it is a bad idea to choose any of these options for your meals.

If you have some busy nights coming up and you need some quick meals that won't keep you in the kitchen half the night, there are a lot of options to choose from. Many people like using an Instant Pot to get things done. Others will pick a slow cooker meal so they can throw the meal in and have it ready when they come home. Freezer meals work great with a plant-based diet. Make any meal that you want and have it ready to pop in the oven when you get home. You just need to pick the method that works the best for you.

Shopping on a plant-based diet is going to change a little bit. You will need to avoid some of the areas that you may have frequented in the past. But with some planning ahead of time and understanding how plant-based nutrition works, you will get used to it and find that it can make your grocery shopping trip easier than before.

Chapter 8: Health Conditions a Plant-Based Diet Can Change

Going on a plant-based diet may have gotten a bad reputation. Many people have chosen to go on more primal diets—ones that really advocate eating a lot of meat and focusing on animal products—while lessening how many carbs you take in. These may not specifically say you need to kick out fruits and vegetables, but they cut down your carb intake, so much that you end up barely getting any in your diet.

Over time, the health of these individuals will go down. They will be hungry all the time. They will take in a lot of bad nutrients into the body and they will miss out on the nutrients they need. This is why a plant-based diet is so important. It makes sure that you are actually able to get all of the nutrients that the body needs, even when you cut down some food groups that aren't the best, without making you feel deprived.

There are a lot of different health conditions that a plant-based diet is able to help with. Spend just a few weeks on it and you will see how amazing it is. Let us see the improvement of some of the health conditions when you decide to adopt a plant-based diet.

Helps in Weight Loss

Many people go on a plant-based diet because they want to lose weight. They may have tried a few different options for weight loss in the past, or they are just starting out and they think this is a great option to help them out. No matter what the reason is, a plant-based diet can help you to lose weight, and in the process, helps you to improve a lot of other health conditions.

Weight loss is simply a matter of eating fewer calories than what is needed to keep up with your daily energy needs. But, following a diet that restricts your calories can be hard. You have to add up your calories, use products that are lower in calories but don't taste good, measure out portions, and feel hungry the whole time. With a plant-based diet, you can really lose weight without all of the hassles of traditional dieting.

One of the big weight loss benefits that you will see in a plant-based diet is the satiety of it. Plant foods have a lot more water in them than your traditional foods. Some examples include:

- Cooked grains have about 70% or more water in them.
- Fresh fruits have about 80% water.
- Root vegetables and potatoes have about 70% water content.
- Green vegetables have more than 90% of water in them.

Now, let's compare these numbers with some of the foods that you may eat on a traditional diet:

- Cooking fats and vegetable oils have 0% water.
- Cornflakes have about 3% water.
- Saltine crackers have 2% water.
- Bagels have 37% water.
- Potato chips have 2% water.

As you can see, the foods that you eat with a plant-based diet have a lot more water in them; and this makes them more filling. Meals that are based on these types of plant foods are more filling, allowing you to eat less and take in fewer calories without feeling deprived all the time. And not only you are eating fewer calories to lose weight, but you are also taking in a ton of nutrients which can assist with weight loss like potassium, antioxidants, vitamin C, vitamin A, and so much more.

So, how well do each of these work? One recent study that was done researched the idea of following a plant-based diet. The subjects were assigned to one out of five diets. These include meat eater, semi-vegetarian, vegetarian but could eat fish, vegetarian, and vegan. None of the participants in this study was told to restrict calories on purpose because researchers wanted to see what would happen naturally.

After two months, the vegetarians and vegans lost the most weight. After two months, all participants could add back some of the foods as they wanted. Even after then, after another four months, the vegetarian and vegans lost twice as much weight as those who were in the other three groups. Out of them all, the group that ate meat lost the least amount of weight.

This helps to show that a plant-based diet is best when it comes to losing weight. Whether you choose to completely get rid of animal products and go vegan or you keep a few in and enjoy dairy and eggs, you are able to lose a lot of weight with these dietary choices.

Helps Build up the Immune System

A plant-based diet can also help you to build up your immune system. Many people have immune systems that are sluggish. They seem to catch everything under the sun and never feel good, especially during the cold and flu season. They may try to take some supplements to help, but these usually don't do a thing and they spend most of the winter on medications just to get through the day.

With a plant-based diet, you are giving the body what it needs to stay healthy and happy. Think about your current animal-based diet. How many fruits and vegetables are you getting in there? The fresh produce that you will enjoy on a plant-based diet has a ton of great nutrients, including vitamin C, which can give your immune system a boost and helps you to feel good and get sick less often than before.

Fights off and Reverses Diabetes

A change in lifestyle and diet can really have an effect on type 2 diabetes. When both are poor, it is the main cause of this disease. But, there is a new research suggesting that vegans are able to reduce their risks of developing diabetes by 79% compared to those who eat animal-based products and meat on a daily basis. As long as the individual follows a vegan diet that is high in fresh produce and low on processed foods and sugar, it is possible to prevent, and sometimes, even fight off diabetes.

For those who eat a plant-based diet, they see a small fraction of the rates of diabetes compared to those who regularly enjoy meat in their meals. By switching to a healthy diet, you could see an improvement in your health, often within a few hours. This is partly due to the fact that vegans are able to control their weight. Carrying around extra body fat is the number one risk factor for type 2 diabetes—at least 90% of those who have diabetes are overweight. Vegans, on the other hand, have lower levels of obesity compared to any other group.

Another issue with the traditional animal product diet is the saturated fats. These fats contribute to insulin resistance, which is a big cause of type 2 diabetes. But when you eat a plant-based diet, you can avoid foods that can cause diabetes, while also eliminating some of the weight that can cause a problem as well.

Can Improve Your Gut Health

If you suffer from gastrointestinal issues, then you may find that a plant-based diet can be the solution that you need. In recent years, researchers have found that there is a big link between gut health and brain health and the rest of the body. Sometimes referred to as the second brain, your stomach is able to affect your immune system, your mood, your memory, how well the body can absorb minerals and vitamins, and basically your overall mental and physical health. But with environmental and dietary stresses that the body encounters, it becomes a struggle for the gut to work properly.

But going on a plant-based diet, especially a vegan one, can have a very positive impact on the health of your gut. A study done in 2015 found that those who ate a Mediterranean diet had a healthier gut compared to those who ate a traditional American diet. In fact, out of the participants in this study, nearly 90% of them were vegan who also adhered to the Mediterranean diet.

While being vegan is not going to cure the gut on its own–you can follow a vegan diet and still eat a bunch of junk–when you combine it with eating a diet that is rich in plants and whole grains, it can work wonders in improving your gut. And once the stomach is able to function properly, the rest of the body will function well too.

Can Protect the Heart

When you go on a plant-based diet, you can help to protect your heart. A diet that is full of animal products often holds more saturated fats and sodium than the body needs. Both of these can make the heart work harder, which can wear you out. The high levels of sodium can be really detrimental to your heart because they can constrict your blood vessels, making the heart work harder to pump nutrients and oxygen to the major organs and causing your blood pressure to rise.

These diets also contain a high level of cholesterol, both in the animal products and in the processed foods you are likely taken in. The body does need to have a bit of cholesterol in it to be healthy. But, you will see cholesterol build up in the arteries of your body when you take in too much of this. If this builds up too much, it can block the arteries, prevent blood from getting to the heart, and cause you to have a heart attack.

When you switch over to a plant-based diet, you can cut out foods that can cause these issues with your heart. You need to cut down on the sodium you consume, as well as on the bad fats and the cholesterol. Instead, you fill the body with lots of fresh produce, which contains the nutrients that the body needs to function properly. Given enough time, you can lower high blood pressure, decrease cholesterol, and more with a plant-based diet.

Can Make the Brain More Focused

When you start to take in all those good nutrients, it can help to focus the mind better. The mind is going to love all the vitamins and minerals it is getting, likely much more than you were getting in the past. The brain needs these nutrients just as much as all the other systems in the body. After just a week on this plant-based diet, you will be able to see the results and you will notice an increase in productivity and mental focus.

In addition to that, when your mind is more focused and is not put down by all that brain fog, you will notice an increase in your energy levels. Those who go on one of these plant-based diets are able to increase their energy levels in no time. You will be able to handle the day better, keep up with the kids, and keep up with more things than ever before.

There are also some primary research that shows how a plant-based diet can help to fight off cognitive disorders like Alzheimer's, and that eating a diet that is rich in fresh produce can even help to lift up your mood, helping with depression and anxiety.

There are so many great benefits that come with a plant-based diet. It can help almost every aspect of your life in terms of health and energy levels. You do not have to be on this plant-based diet very long before you notice all the great benefits that come with it.

Chapter 9: Bonus Chapter – Healthy Recipe Ideas

Peanut Butter and Chocolate Smoothie

What's inside:

Water (1 cup)
Non-dairy milk of choice (.5 cup)
Spinach (1 cup)
Maple syrup (1 tbsp.)
Peanut butter (1 tbsp.)
Unsweetened cocoa powder (1 tbsp.)
Chia seeds (1 tbsp.)
Rolled oats (.25 cup)
Banana (1)

How to make:

1. Bring out your blender and puree everything together. Add in some more milk if you want a smoother consistency.
2. Serve in four cups when you are done.

Breakfast Oatmeal Cookies

What's inside:

Raisins (.25 cup)
Rolled oats (.5 cup)
Salt
Nutmeg (.25 tsp.)
Ground cinnamon (1 tsp.)
Banana, mashed (1)
Maple syrup (2 tbsp.)
Almond butter (2 tbsp.)
Ground flaxseed (1 tbsp.)

How to make:

1. Turn on the oven and give it time to heat up to 350°F. Take a baking sheet and line it with some parchment paper.
2. Mix together the flaxseed with 3 tablespoons of water. Leave it to sit.
3. In another bowl, mix together the maple syrup and almond butter until it is creamy. Add in the banana. Then, add in your flaxseed and water mixture.
4. Sift the salt, nutmeg, and cinnamon into a bowl and then stir it in with the wet mixture. Add in the raisins and oats and fold it in.
5. Form these into small balls and then press onto a baking sheet. Place into the oven to bake.
6. Bake for 12 minutes to make golden brown. Serve or store properly.

Applesauce Muffins

What's inside:

Walnuts, chopped (.5 cup)
Salt
Cinnamon (1 tsp.)
Baking powder (.5 tsp.)
Baking soda (1 tsp.)
Whole grain flour (2 cups)
Vanilla (1 tsp.)
Apple cider vinegar (1 tsp.)
Flaxseed (2 tbsp.)
Non-dairy milk (.5 cup)
Coconut sugar (.33 cup)
Unsweetened applesauce (1.5 cups)
Nut butter (2 tbsp.)
Coconut oil (1 tsp.)

How to make:

1. Turn on the oven and let it heat up to 350°F. Get two muffin tins ready by greasing it with some coconut oil.
2. In a bowl, mix together the vanilla, vinegar, flaxseed, milk, coconut sugar, applesauce, and nut butter.
3. In another bowl, sift together the chopped walnuts, salt, cinnamon, baking powder, baking soda, and flour.
4. Mix together the wet ingredients and dry ingredients until they are combined.

5. Spoon some of this batter into each muffin cup. Place into the oven to bake.
6. After 15 minutes, the applesauce muffins should be done. Allow them to cool down before serving.

Hearty Chili

What's inside:

Cilantro (.25 cup)
Salt (.25 tsp.)
Chili powder (3 tsp.)
Kidney beans (1 can)
Tomato paste (.25 cup)
Tomatoes (1 can)
Olive oil (1 tsp.)
Garlic cloves, minced (2)
Onion, diced (1)

How to make:

1. Bring out a big pot and sauté the garlic and onion in oil for 5 minutes. Once these are soft, add in the chili powder, beans, tomato paste, and tomatoes. Season with some salt.
2. Let these ingredients simmer for 10 minutes, or as long as you need them to.
3. Garnish with some cilantro, then serve.

Creamy Pumpkin Soup

What's inside:

Pepper
Walnuts, toasted (.25 cup)
Non-dairy milk (1 cup)
Nutritional yeast (3 tbsp.)
Ground sage (3 tsp.)
Water (4 cups)
Onion, diced (1)
Salt (.25 tsp.)
Olive oil (1 tsp.)
Pumpkin (1)

How to make:

1. Bring out a pan and heat it up before cooking the pumpkin in the oil. Season with some salt and let it cook until it becomes soft, after 10 minutes.
2. Add in the onion and let it cook for another five minutes.
3. Add in the water. Bring it to a boil, then reduce to a simmer.
4. Put the lid on and let these all cook for the next 20 minutes, or until the pumpkin is tender.
5. Stir in the milk, nutritional yeast, and the sage. Using an immersion blender, puree the soup until it is smooth.
6. Garnish soup with some pepper and the toasted walnuts before you serve.

Moroccan Salad

What's inside:

Spinach, chopped (2 cups)
Mint, chopped
Garlic clove, pressed (1)
Green olives, chopped (1 tbsp.)
Capers (2 tbsp.)
Lemon, half juiced and half zested
Salt
Nutmeg (.25 tsp.)
Turmeric (.25 tsp.)
Ground ginger (.5 tsp.)
Cumin (.5 tsp.)
Eggplant, diced (1)
Olive oil (1 tsp.)

How to make:

1. Heat up some oil in a skillet, then add in the eggplant. Once the eggplant softened a bit, stir in the turmeric, ginger, cumin, salt, and nutmeg.
2. Cook this for another 10 minutes to make the eggplant nice and soft.
3. After this time, add in the mint, garlic, olives, capers, lemon juice, and zest. Cook for a few more minutes.
4. Add a few handfuls of spinach on the plate and then spoon the eggplant on top. Serve right away.

Dill Potato Salad

What's inside:

Chives, chopped (1 tbsp.)
Red bell pepper (1)
Celery stalks, chopped (3)
Non-dairy milk
Nutritional yeast (1 tbsp.)
Pepper
Salt
Dijon mustard (2 tsp.)
Dill, chopped (.25 cup)
Zucchini, chopped (1)
Potatoes, chopped (6)

How to make:

1. Bring out a pot and fill it up about a quarter of the way with some water. Let the water boil before adding in the potatoes.
2. Boil potatoes for 10 minutes.
3. Add in the zucchini and let it cook for another 10 minutes. After that time, take these out of the pot and drain out, saving about a cup of the liquid. Let the vegetable set in a bowl to cool down.
4. Take half a cup of the potatoes and move them over to a blender with the reserved liquid. Add in the nutritional yeast, pepper, salt, mustard, and dill.
5. Puree these until smooth. Add a bit of non-dairy milk if you need it to be a little smoother.

6. Take out a bowl and toss in the cooked potatoes, chives, bell pepper, celery, and zucchini. Pour the dressing on top and then toss around to coat.

Curry Lentil Burgers

What's inside:

Pepper
Salt
Curry powder (2 tsp.)
Whole grain flour (.75 cup)
Onion, chopped (1)
Carrots, grated (3)
Water (3 cups)
Lentils (1 cup)

How to make:

1. Put the lentils into a pot with some water. Let the water come to a boil and then simmer this for the next 30 minutes until soft.
2. While your lentils are cooking, put the chopped onion and grated carrots in a bowl. Toss them with the pepper, salt, curry powder, and flour.
3. When the lentils are done, drain off the extra water and throw them in with the veggies. Use a potato masher to mash this up a bit, and add more flour to get the mixture to stick together.
4. Using your hands, make 12 patties out of this mixture, adding in the amount of flour that you need.
5. Heat up a large skillet with a bit of oil and place the patties in. Cook them for 10 minutes on one side. Flip them over and cook for another 5 minutes before serving.

Loaded Pizza

What's inside:

Avocado, sliced (1)
Red onion, sliced (1)
Salt
Carrot, grated (1)
Pepper
Tomato, sliced (1)
Spicy black bean dip (.5 cup)
Pizza crust, prebaked (2)

How to make:

1. Turn on the oven and heat it up to 400°F. Lay out the crusts onto a baking sheet. Spread half the bean dip onto each crust and then layer on the tomato and avocado slices.
2. Sprinkle the grated carrots and some salt on top of the prepared crusts.
3. Add the onion on top of it all.
4. Place this into the oven and let it bake. After 15 minutes, the pizzas should be done and you can serve.

Pad Thai Bowl

What's inside:

Fresh lime wedges
Peanuts, roasted (2 tbsp.)
Cilantro, chopped (.25 cup)
Peanut sauce (.25 cup)
Bean sprouts (1 cup)
Mint, chopped (3 tbsp.)
Scallions, chopped (2)
Red bell pepper, sliced (1)
Red cabbage, sliced (1 cup)
Carrots, julienned (2)
Olive oil (1 tsp.)
Brown rice noodles (7 oz.)

How to make:

1. Put the rice noodles into a pot of boiling water and let these set for 10 minutes so they become tender. Rinse, drain, and then set it aside to cool down.
2. Heat up some oil in a skillet. Add the cabbage, carrots, and bell pepper.
3. After 8 minutes, toss in the bean sprouts, mint, and scallions. Cook for a few more minutes before removing all these from the stove.
4. Toss the noodles with the vegetables and then top with the peanut sauce.
5. Add these to your serving bowls and sprinkle with the peanuts and cilantro. Serve with a lime wedge and enjoy.

Taco Salad Bowl

What's inside:

Black Bean Salad
Scallions, chopped (2)
Red bell pepper, chopped (1)
Cherry tomatoes (1.5 cups)
Salt
Chili powder (2 tsp.)
Juice from one lime
Cilantro, chopped (.25 cup)
Corn kernels (1 c.)
Black beans (1 can)

1 Serving of Tortilla Chips
Pepper
Salt
Olive oil (1 tsp.)
Whole grain wrap or tortilla (1)
Chili powder
Dried oregano

For One Bowl
Mango salsa (.25 cup)
Avocado, chopped (.25 cup)
Quinoa or brown rice, cooked (.75 cup)
Fresh greens (1 cup)

How to make:

1. Start with the black bean salad. To do this, just toss all the ingredients together in a bowl.
2. Now, you can make the tortilla chips. Brush your tortilla with some olive oil and sprinkle on the chili powder, oregano, pepper, and salt.
3. Slice this into 8 pieces like a pizza and put them to a baking sheet. Turn the oven on to 400°F and put the tortilla chips inside.
4. After 5 minutes, take them out and give them some time to cool down before moving on.
5. Now, make the bowl. Lay the greens inside the bowl and top with the cooked quinoa or brown rice, the tortilla chips, a third of the black bean salad, the salsa, and the avocado before serving.

Almond Energy Bites

What's inside:

Cocoa nibs (.25 cup)
Almonds, ground (.75 cup)
Chia seeds (.25 cup)
Shredded coconut (1 cup)
Dates, pitted (1 cup)

How to make:

1. Take all the ingredients and add them into a food processor, pureeing them until they would stick together.
2. Form this mixture into 24 balls and then place them onto a baking sheet that has a parchment paper.
3. Put these inside the fridge and let them sit for 15 minutes before serving.

Coconut and Mango Cream Pie

What's inside:

The Crust
Soft pitted dates (1 cup)
Cashews (1 cup)
Rolled oats (.5 cup)

For the Filling
Shredded coconut (.5 cup)
Mangoes, chopped and peeled (2)
Water (.5 cup)
Canned coconut milk (1 cup)

How to make:

1. Put all of the ingredients for the crust into the food processor. Pulse until they start to hold together.
2. Take this mixture and press it down firmly into a pie pan.
3. Put all of your filling ingredients into a blender. Puree these until they are smooth. You want this to be thick, so you may have to stop and stir it all around.
4. Pour this filling into the crust, and use a rubber spatula to smoothen the top a bit.
5. Put the pie inside the freezer. Let it sit for about 30 minutes. Serve when ready.

Avocado and Blueberry Cheesecake

What's inside:

For the Crust
Lime zest (1 tsp.)
Soft pitted dates (1 cup)
Walnuts (1 cup)
Rolled oats (1 cup)

For the Filling
Basil, minced (2 tbsp.)
Lime juice (4 tbsp.)
Maple syrup (2 tbsp.)
Blueberries (1 cup)
Avocados, pitted (2)

How to make:

1. Put all of the crust ingredients into the food processor and pulse until well-combined.
2. Take this mixture and press it down into a pie pan, pushing into the bottom or along the sides.
3. Take all your ingredients for the filling and add them to a blender. Puree on high until smooth.
4. Pour the filling into the crust. Use a spatula to help smoothen the top and make it even.
5. Put the cheesecake inside the freezer. Let it set for 2-3 hours before serving.

Chocolate Banana Cupcakes

What's inside:

Dark chocolate chips (.25 cup)
Salt
Chia seeds (.25 cup)
Unsweetened cocoa powder (.5 cup)
Baking soda (.5 tsp.)
Baking powder (1 tsp.)
Coconut sugar (.25 cup)
Rolled oats (.5 cup)
Whole-grain flour (1.25 cup)
Pure vanilla (1 tsp.)
Apple cider vinegar (1 tsp.)
Almond butter (2 tbsp.)
Non-dairy milk (1 cup)
Bananas (3)

How to make:

1. Turn on the oven and give it time to heat up to 350°F. Prepare two muffin tins with some paper cups in it.
2. Add the vanilla, vinegar, almond butter, milk, and bananas in a blender and puree until smooth. You can also stir these together in a bowl to make them creamy and smooth.
3. In a separate bowl, pour all the dry ingredients together— sugar, baking powder, oats, flour, chocolate chips, salt, chia seeds, cocoa powder, and baking soda. Stir to combine these well.

4. When this is done, mix the dry and the wet ingredients together. Stir to combine the mixture. Spoon this mixture into the muffin cups and then place these into the oven and bake for about 20 minutes.
5. Once done, take them out of the oven and give them time to cool down a bit before serving.

Conclusion

A plant-based diet can be a great program to follow. It helps you to get back to the basics, back to feeding your body the exact nutrients that it needs without all the added extras that can make you sick or can ruin your health. It goes against the rules that come with a traditional American diet, but all the benefits make it worth the time and effort to follow it.

Many people may feel that a plant-based diet is just a vegetarian diet or a vegan diet. While these two diet plans fall under the idea of plant-based nutrition, the ideas behind why people follow each one can be different. Many of those who follow plant-based nutrition program are not as concerned with the environment, although some are. They are concerned about doing what is best for their health. And through the many studies out there, they have found that a plant-based diet is the best way to give their bodies lots of energy and nutrients that help them to fight off chronic illnesses and other diseases.

This guidebook has spent some time looking at the benefits of going on a plant-based diet. We have discussed how the typical omnivore diet can really mess with your health and that eating plant-based food can really make a difference in how you feel overall. This is such a simple program, one that many people throughout the world have already discovered, and you can use it for your own benefit as well!

When you are ready to improve your health and you want to reduce your risk or eliminate chronic illness in your life and just want to have more energy, then, plant-based nutrition is the best solution for you. This guidebook will give you the information that you need to get started!

Here, we have discussed what plant-based nutrition is, the health benefits it can help you with, what types of food you should consume, and the best way to hit the grocery store to stick with this nutrition idea.